MEDITERRANEAN DIET COOKBOOK

200+ Tasty Recipes

To stay healthy and reach your ideal weight. Your decisive choice for eating and living well

Antonio Fiorucci

Table of Contents

INTRODUCTION.............................9

ABOUT THE MEDITERRANEAN DIET 15

Benefits of the Mediterranean Diet 15

Mediterranean Diet Pyramid 16

THE MEDITERRANEAN FOOD PYRAMID....... 19

WHAT TO EAT: THE MEDITERRANEAN DIET
FOOD LIST 22

What you can eat 22

Food to Avoid 23

COMMON MISTAKES 25

EATING OUT ON THE MEDITERRANEAN DIET
.... 28

GETTING STARTED WITH THE
MEDITERRANEAN DIET AND MEAL PLANNING
.... 33

Planning Your Mediterranean Diet 33

BREAKFAST.................................. 37

Caprese Poached Eggs 38

Sautéed Greens and Eggs.........................39

Breakfast Pizza 40

Caprese on Sourdough..........................42

Mediterranean Inspired Breakfast Quinoa 43

Eggs Florentine.......................................44

Egg White Breakfast Sandwich 46

Mediterranean Egg Wrap 47

Quinoa Bowl 48

Yogurt Figs Mix 50

Seeds and Lentils Oats................................... 51

Cinnamon Apple and Lentils Porridge...................52

Coriander Mushroom Salad...............................54

Feta Baked Eggs..55

Banana Oats 56

Berry Oats 57

Muesli and Fresh Fruits Oatmeal.........................58

Quinoa Muffins 59

Greek Cheesy Yogurt 60

Walnuts Yogurt Mix 61

Tahini Pine Nuts Toast.....................................62

Raspberries and Yogurt Smoothie 63

Cottage Cheese and Berries Omelet 64

Banana Cinnamon Fritters...................................65

French Toast..66

Chocolat Quinoa Porridge 67

Greedy Rice Milk 68

PASTA 69

Mediterranean Diet White Bean & Tomato Pasta . 70

Shrimp Scampi 71

Lighter Lasagna 72

Greek Pasta Salad 73

Insalata Caprese II Salad 75

Chopped Israeli Mediterranean Pasta Salad 76

Seafood Linguine 77

Spaghetti Squash with Shrimp Scampi 78

Cajun Seafood Pasta 80

Tortellini in Red Pepper Sauce 81

Linguine and Brussels Sprouts 82

Creamy Chickpea Sauce with Whole-Wheat Fusilli 84

SOUPS RECIPES 85

Roasted Pepper Soup 86

Italian Meatball Soup 87

Tuscan White Bean Soup with Sausage and Kale ... 88

Vegetable Soup 90

Moroccan Lentil Soup 92

Roasted Red Pepper and Tomato Soup 94

Greek Spring Soup 95

Minestrone Soup 96

Lemon Chicken Soup 98

Tuscan Vegetable Pasta Soup 99

Avgolemono Soup 101

Italian Wedding Soup 102

Lentil and Beef Soup 103

Beef and Vegetable Soup 105

Beef and Vegetable Minestrone 106

Bean, Chicken and Sausage Soup 107

Moroccan Chicken and Butternut Squash Soup... 108

Chicken Soup with Vermicelli 110

MEAT RECIPES 113

Crockpot Beef Stroganoff 114

Pork Stew with Oyster Mushrooms..................... 115

Easy Crockpot Pork Loin 116

Braised Short Ribs with Red Wine 117

Lamb Kofte with Yogurt Sauce 118

Mediterranean Pork Roast 119

Beef, Artichoke & Mushroom Stew 121

Beef & Tapioca Stew 123

Beef Pizza... 125

Beef & Bulgur Meatballs 127

Tasty Beef and Broccoli 129

Beef Corn Chili 130

Balsamic Beef Dish 131

Soy Sauce Beef Roast 133

Rosemary Beef Chuck Roast 134

Pork Chops and Tomato Sauce: 135

Pork Potato 136

Coffee Flavored Pork Ribs 138

Tomato Pork Paste 139

Garlic Pulled Pork 140

Buttered Pork Chops 142

Quick and Easy Pork Loin Roast 143

Cheese and Ham Roll-ups 144

Meat Cup Snacks 146

Pork and Cheese Stuffed Peppers 147

Peppered Pork Rack 148

Pork Belly 150

Easy Pork Chops 151

Coffee BBQ Pork Belly 152

Mustard and Rosemary Pork Tenderloin 153

Stuffed Pork Loin with Sun-Dried Tomato and Goat Cheese 155

Flank Steak with Orange-Herb Pistou 157

Beef Kofta 159

Spicy Beef with Olives and Feta 161

Best Ever Beef Stew 162

One Pot Mediterranean Spiced Beef and Macaroni 164

Beef and Cheese Gratin 166

Beef Cacciatore 167

Greek Beef and Veggie Skewers 168

Pork Tenderloin with Orzo 170

Grilled Pork Chops with Tomato Salad 171

Boneless Pork Chops with Summer Veggies 172

One Skillet Mediterranean Pork and Rice 174

Garlic and Rosemary Mediterranean Pork Roast . 176

Pork Tenderloin with Roasted Vegetables 177

SEAFOOD RECIPES 179

Crockpot Garlic and Shrimps 180

Roasted Red Snapper 181

Healthy Carrot & Shrimp 182

Salmon with Potatoes 184

Honey Garlic Shrimp 185

Pan-Fried Cod 186

Simple Lemon Clams 187

Grilled Marinated Shrimp 188

Grilled Salmon 190

Cedar Planked Salmon 191

Broiled Tilapia Parmesan 192

Fish Tacos 194

Grilled Tilapia with Mango Salsa 196

Blackened Salmon Fillets 198

Seafood Enchiladas 200

Seafood Stuffing 202

Scrumptious Salmon Cakes 203

Easy Tuna Patties 204

Heather's Grilled Salmon 206

Brown Butter Perch 207

APPETIZERS 209

Greek Yogurt (Used as Dip) 210

Lemon Garlic Sesame Hummus Dip 211

Creamy Greek Yogurt and Cucumber ... 212

Nachos 213

Stuffed Celery 214

Butternut Squash Fries 215

Dried Fig Tapenade 216

Speedy Sweet Potato Chips 217

Nachos with Hummus (Mediterranean Inspired) . 218

Pineapple Mediterranean Dip 220

Mediterranean Inspired Tapenade 221

Hummus and Olive Pita Bread 222

Lime Yogurt Dip 223

Chicken Kale Wraps 224

VEGETARIAN 225

Italian Style Roasted Vegetables 226

Mediterranean Diet Lemon Kale 227

Chickpeas and Millet Stew 229

Crispy Black-Eyed Peas 230

Lemony Green Beans 231

Roasted Orange Cauliflower 232

Eggplant Parmesan Panini 234

Spinach Samosa 236

Avocado Fries 237

Potato Tortilla with Leeks and Mushrooms 238

Creamy Sweet Potatoes and Collards ... 240

Roasted Vegetables and Chickpeas 242

Veggie Rice Bowls with Pesto Sauce 244

VEGETABLES 247

Quinoa with Almonds and Cranberries 248

Mediterranean Baked Chickpeas 249

Falafel Bites 250

Quick Vegetable Kebabs 252

Freekeh, Chickpea, and Herb Salad 253

Mediterranean Farro Bowl 254

Mozzarella and Sun-Dried Portobello Mushroom Pizza 255

Honey Roasted Carrots 257

SIDES AND SALADS 259

Bacon Cheddar Broccoli Salad 260

Peppers and Lentils Salad 261

Cashews and Red Cabbage Salad 262

Apples and Pomegranate Salad 263

Cranberry Bulgur Mix 265

Chickpeas, Corn and Black Beans Salad...............266

Olives and Lentils Salad 267

Lime Spinach and Chickpeas Salad 268

Minty Olives and Tomatoes Salad......................269

Beans and Cucumber Salad................................270

Tomato and Avocado Salad 272

Arugula Salad 273

Chickpea Salad..274

Feta Tomato Salad...275

Lebanese Lentil Salad with Garlic & Herbs 277

Lime & Honey Fruit Salad 278

POULTRY 279

Italian Chicken with Zucchini Noodles 280

Chicken and Kale Tortilla Stew..........................281

Sticky Chicken Wings 282

Lemon Grass and Coconut Chicken Drumsticks....284

Lemon-Rosemary Spatchcock Chicken 285

Chicken Yellow Curry...................................287

Caprese-Stuffed Chicken Breasts 289

Chicken with Caper Sauce 291

Chicken Stuffed Peppers 293

Italian Chicken...295

Lemon Garlic Chicken 297

Chicken with Salsa & Cilantro 298

Chicken & Rice..300

Chicken Skillet 302

Chicken Shawarma 304

Mediterranean Chicken 306

Lime Chicken with Black Beans..........................307

Mediterranean Chicken Wings 308

Honey Balsamic Chicken 310

Turkey Verde with Brown Rice 311

Turkey with Basil & Tomatoes...........................312

DESSERTS 315

Butter Pie 316

Homemade Spinach Pie....................................317

Blueberries Bowls 318

Rhubarb Strawberry Crunch 319

Banana Dessert with Chocolate Chips 320

Cranberry and Pistachio Biscotti.........................321

Minty Watermelon Salad 322

Mascarpone and Fig Crostini 324

Crunchy Sesame Cookies 325

Almond Cookies 326

Baklava and Honey 328

Date and Nut Balls 330

Creamy Rice Pudding 332

Ricotta-Lemon Cheesecake 334

Crockpot Keto Chocolate Cake 335

Keto Crockpot Chocolate Lava Cake 336

Lemon Crockpot Cake 338

Lemon and Watermelon Granita 339

Baked Apples with Walnuts and Spices 340

Red Wine Poached Pears 342

Vanilla Pudding with Strawberries 343

Mixed Berry Frozen Yogurt Bar 345

Vanilla Cream 346

Brownies 347

Strawberries Coconut Cake 349

Cocoa Almond Pudding 350

Nutmeg Cream 352

Vanilla Avocado Cream 353

Raspberries Cream Cheese Bowls 354

Mediterranean Watermelon Salad 356

Coconut Apples 357

Orange Compote 358

Pears Stew 359

Lemon Watermelon Mix 360

Rhubarb Cream 361

Mango Bowls 362

Chocolate Ganache 364

Chocolate Covered Strawberries 365

Strawberry Angel Food Dessert 366

Fruit Pizza 368

Bananas Foster 370

Cranberry Orange Cookies 371

Introduction

The Mediterranean diet is a diet developed in the United States in the 1980s and inspired by Italy and Greece's eating habits in the 1960s. This diet's main aspects include proportionally high intake of olive oil, nuts and seeds, unprocessed cereals, fruits, veggies, moderate to high fish consumption, and regular drinking of dairy products (mostly as cheese and yogurt). Olive oil has been known as a potential health factor in reducing mortality from all causes and the risk of chronic diseases.

The Mediterranean diet has been proven to be an excellent way of maintaining health and living a long, healthy life. It is undoubtedly a great diet plan to follow. The Italian Mediterranean diet can also create long-term effects in keeping one's heart-healthy and body functioning at optimum levels. That is why the American Medical Association and the (AHA) American Heart Association suggest this diet.

Mediterranean Diet is a lifestyle more than a mere diet. It's safe to say the Mediterranean diet is both a brain-friendly and a body-friendly diet because it preserves and keeps them balanced in their respective ways. Therefore, as long as you follow this Mediterranean diet and continue to enrich your lifestyle with the balanced meal options it provides, you are assured of leading a safe and wonderful life without diseases hiding nearby.

Brief History of Italian Cuisine

The first traces of Italian cuisine date back to ancient times, when Sicily was among the Roman Empire's most important provinces. Then, when the Roman Empire fell, in AD 476, Sicily was occupied by the Ostrogoths for 300 years, unlike most of Italy's rest. During this time, some of the earliest cookbooks for cooking, Apicius, was written. Apicius and other cookbooks played a role in passing on to successive generations the cooking traditions of antiquity. Salvius was a chef who lived around 400 and a half centuries ago. His cooking was done in what was called the kitchen of gastronomy. It was a place where chefs of the Imperial Court gathered. Some recipes found in Apicius are very elaborate. Another essential cookbook from this period is De Re Coquinaria; Maestro Martino wrote this. This cookbook contains elements of Arab, Moorish, and Northern European cooking.

The first Italian cookbook written in 1472 is known as a book of the table's pleasures. This cookbook did not give measurements to the directions for the recipes. Instead, it included many different versions of ingredients and flavors.

In 1475, Fornaio was written by a person named Bartolomeo Sacchi, known as Platina. This book was the first cookbook written in the Italian language. It contained around 250 recipes that involved the measurement of the ingredients.

Platina described the different meals to be served. Platina included the proper foods to serve, such as the right ingredients to buy from a market and the foods that should be avoided. The recipes were very elaborate and complicated. In this book, there were numerous rules about food preparation, how many dishes should be ready for a meal, how many guests to serve, and how to serve and clean up after the meal.

Around 1570, the Book of Cooking by Bartolomeo Scappi was written. Plinio il Vecchio (Gaius Plinius Secundus) is the first cooking author to mention olive oil in his recipes. It helped to develop the beginning of the first cookbook by Bartol Omeo Scappi. He was an Italian monk and scientist from Padua, Italy. In 1570, he became the private cook for the powerful Medici family in Florence, Italy. He started to work and create recipes for them. His cookbook was written to help give the Medici family a reputation of being wealthy and sophisticated.

This cookbook mainly contained recipes for desserts, sweets, and different types of cocktails. A variety of meats and vegetables were used in these recipes, including many kinds of seafood. Many of the fruits in these recipes were imported from different countries such as Turkey and Sicily. There were a lot of ingredients and recipes that were imported from other countries as well. The book included around 400 recipes. He also had instructions on how to make different dishes.

Many of the recipes were based on different ones from around Europe. He made simple Italian recipes for more complicated dishes. For example, he used a chicken breast and then took fat pork belly and added it to the meat." Scappi also had a recipe for rabbit stuffed with bacon and chicken pigeons tied with leeks." It is an example of how he would change an already high dish and make it even higher. There is a difference between these high-class recipes and lower-class recipes. The high-class recipes were more complicated and more entertaining. The low-class recipes were less extravagant.

For the food, the dishes had only one main course. It was a sit-down dinner or an important meal. They had many different types of bread and desserts to choose from. The bread and bread products were made of many different grains and types of flour. The bread was the primary source of food in the lower classes.

Along with bread, the people had boiled greens and boiled meats. The greens were cooked with vinegar and butter-based sauce. The meats were boiled in water with salt. The meats were boiled and put into something to make it easier to eat. They had a different type of meat called frassetto, similar to beef, but it was more tender. Other meats were also consumed. The meat was slowly roasted in an oven called a spit. All classes liked the bread. People from every social class were able to buy and enjoy the bread.

The ingredients that the people used was essential. The vegetables included onions, leeks, escarole, cabbage, beans, Romano beans, carrots, lettuce, garlic, and legume. The basic types of cheese were mozzarella, Parmesan, ricotta, butter cheese from Tuscany, and sheep's cheese. Baked goods included butter cakes, puff pastry cakes, and cakes made of apricots, dates, and nuts. The wine included certain types made in Sicily. The drinks included mead, honeyed, and carob drinks, and the meats included beef, veal, mutton, pork, wild boar, goat, goose, chicken, duck, geese, and partridge.

The food wasn't the only thing of importance. The way that the food was served and the decor was important too. The hosts of these dinners and the guests had to dress up as well. The guests wore unique clothes; the women wore silk, velvet, and cotton velvets, and the men also wore silk and velvet. The tableware was usually made of gold, silver, and porcelain. They also used wood that was overlaid with the mother of pearl. It was used by the wealthier people who didn't need to decorate their tableware.

The food of the middle class was a little different from the upper class. The middle class had food with an emphasis on herbs, such as sage, rosemary, and mint. The middle class cooked plainer foods and mainly used grains. The foods that the middle class served were used to entertain guests and also for dinner. The dinner was the more formal meal of the day.

As Italy's food started to change and develop, so did the rooms and space used to serve the food. Initially, they would use the kitchen and the dining room in one area. There were no separate rooms for cooking and eating in Italy. After this style, the French style came around. This style had many rooms. The rooms were a big deal because they created more organization for the service of the food. The rooms were called the entrée, the cellar, the pantry, the scullery, the larder, the kitchen, the meat larder, the pastry room, and the servant's bedroom. The meat larder and the larder were the most important parts of the kitchen.

In the larder, the food was kept and cooked. In the meat, the larder was where the meat was kept cold. The room had a window so that the cold air could come through and keep the food cold. The larders are usually dark and low. The shape of the room is rectangular. The room is generally in the shape of a desk. The food is kept on a shelf that is built into the room. In a lot of larders, there is no electricity. It means that the food and food products can't be kept as cold. The larders are either fake or real. It is common for fake larders to be created in apartments.

The food served to the Italian people was very diverse, and it changed as many cultures influenced it. Some of these cultures were Chinese, early Indian, and Turkish. Each culture influenced the food and the way that the food was prepared. Also, as new cultures were introduced to Italy, the food changed with it.

Some of these cultures are known to us, and they, in turn, had their own cuisine. Other cultures stayed out of the public eye, and there is not much known about them that is useful. These cultures are all known, and there is more information available. The Turks were Italian allies in the sixteenth century, so there was a lot of trade between Turkey and Italy.

There are also Arab and Chinese influences that were not as well documented. Arab cuisine was developed in Italy as well.

In the 15th century, a new concept of food from this area was introduced. A strong Italian influence on cooking was created, and Justin Barrett wrote the book Cooking with Grease. In the 20th century, the Italian Mediterranean diet's essential elements were established, including a high intake of vegetables, fruit, and olive oil. However, the cuisine itself was not as refined as it is today. Before the mid-19th century, food often consisted of essential vegetable and meat stews and casseroles.

It is essential to know that the Italian Mediterranean diet now is a safe stronghold for us to hold onto and make it known to people to lead a healthy life. Nonetheless, its disappearance is a real danger and a threat to the good society we have long worked for and envisaged.

About the Mediterranean Diet

The Mediterranean diet is full of never-ending varieties of healthy, fresh, and delicious foods. However, there is more of an emphasis on certain types of foods, nothing is excluded. People who try a Mediterranean diet can enjoy the dishes they love while also learning to appreciate how good the freshest, healthiest foods can be.

Transitioning into the Mediterranean diet is mainly about bracing yourself for a new way of eating, adapting your attitude toward food into one of joyful expectation and appreciation of good meals and good company. It's like a mindset as anything else, so you'll want to make your environment unite so you can quickly adapt to the lifestyle in the Mediterranean way.

Benefits of the Mediterranean Diet

Boosts Your Brain Health: Preserve memory and prevent cognitive decline by following the Mediterranean diet that will limit processed foods, refined bread, and red meats. Have a glass of wine versus hard liquor.

Improves Poor Eyesight: Older individuals suffer from poor eyesight, but in many cases, the Mediterranean diet has provided notable improvement. An Australian Center for Eye Research discovered that the individuals who consumed a minimum of 100 ml (0.42 cup) of olive oil weekly were almost 50% less likely to develop macular degeneration versus those who ate less than one ml each week.

Helps to Reduce the Risk of Heart Disease: The New England Journal of Medicine provided evidence in 2013 from a randomized clinical trial. The trial was implemented in Spain, whereas individuals did not have cardiovascular disease at enrollment but were in the 'high risk' category. The incidence of major cardiovascular events was reduced by the Mediterranean diet that was supplemented with extra-virgin olive oil or nuts. In one study, men who consumed fish in this manner reduced the risk by 23% of death from heart disease.

The Risk of Alzheimer's disease is reduced: In 2018, the journal Neurology studied 70 brain scans of individuals who had no signs of dementia at the onset. They followed the eating patterns in a two-year study resulting in individuals who were on the Med diet had a lesser increase of the depots and reduced energy use - potentially signaling risk for Alzheimer's.

Helps Lessen the Risk of Some Types of Cancer: According to the results of a group study, the diet is associated with a lessened risk of stomach cancer (gastric adenocarcinoma).

Decreases Risks for Type 2 Diabetes: It can help stabilize blood sugar while protecting against type 2 diabetes with its low-carb elements. The Med diet maintains a richness in fiber, which will digest slowly while preventing variances in your blood sugar. It also can help you maintain a healthier weight, which is another trigger for diabetes.

Suggests Improvement for Those with Parkinson's disease: By consuming foods on the Mediterranean diet, you add high levels of antioxidants that can prevent your body from undergoing oxidative stress, which is a damaging process that will attack your cells. The menu plan can reduce your risk factors in half.

Mediterranean Diet Pyramid

The Mediterranean Diet Pyramid is a nutritional guide developed by the World Health Organization, Harvard School of Public Health, and Oldways Preservation Trust in 1993. It is a visual tool that summarizes the Mediterranean diet, suggested eating patterns, and guides how frequently specific mechanisms should be eaten. It allows you to break healthy eating habits and not overfill yourself with too many calories.

Olive oil, fruits, vegetables, whole grains, legumes, beans, nuts & seeds, spices & herbs: These foods form the Mediterranean pyramid base. If you did observe, you would notice that these are mostly from plant sources. You should try and include a few variations of these items into each meal you eat. Olive oil should be the primary fat in cooking your dishes and endeavor to replace any other butter or cooking oil you may have been using to cook.

Fish & seafood: These are essential staples of the Mediterranean diet that should be consumed often as a protein source. You would want to include these in your diet at least two times a week. Try new varieties of fish, either frozen or fresh. Also, incorporate seafood like mussels, crab, and shrimp into your diet. Canned tuna is also great to include on sandwiches or toss in a salad with fresh vegetables.

Cheese, yogurt, eggs & poultry: These ingredients should be consumed in more moderate amounts. Depending on the food, they should be used sparingly throughout the week. Keep in mind that if you are using eggs in baking or cooking, they will also be counted in your weekly limit. You would want to stick to more healthy cheese like Parmesan, ricotta, or feta that you can add a topping or garnish on your dishes.

Red meat & sweets: These items are going to be consumed less frequently. If you are going to eat them, you need to consume only small quantities, most preferably lean meat versions with less fat when possible. Most studies recommend a maximum of 12 to 16 ounces per month. To add more variety to your diet, you can still have red meat occasionally, but you would want to reduce how often you have it. It is essential to limit its intake because of all the health concerns of sugar and red meat. The Mediterranean diet improves cardiovascular health and reduces blood pressure, while red meat tends to be dangerous to your cardiovascular system. The Greece population ate very little red meat and instead had fish or seafood as their main protein source.

Water: The Mediterranean diet encourages you to stay hydrated at all times. It means drinking more water than your daily intake. The Institute of Medicine recommends a total of 9 cups each day for women and 13 cups for men. For pregnant or breastfeeding women, the number should be increased.

Wine: Moderate consumption of wine with meals is encouraged on the Mediterranean diet. Studies shown that moderate consumption of alcohol can reduce the risk of heart disease. That can mean about 1 glass per day for women. Men tend to have higher body mass so that they can consume 1 to 2 drinks. Please keep in mind what your doctor would recommend regarding wine consumption based on your health and family history.

The Mediterranean Food Pyramid

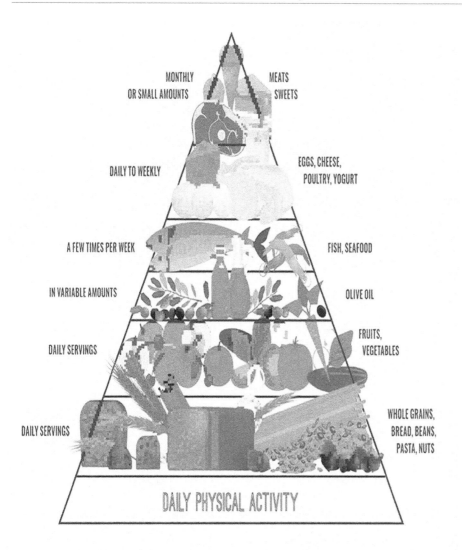

The Mediterranean Diet Pyramid is a visual tool that summarizes the Mediterranean Diet's suggested pattern of eating and gives a guide to how frequently specific tools should be eaten. This allows you to have a breakdown of healthy eating habits and not overfill yourself with too many calories.

How is the pyramid laid out? Let's go over each tier.

Olive oil, fruits, vegetables, whole grains, legumes, beans, nuts & seeds, spices & herbs: These are the types of food that form the base of the Mediterranean pyramid. You'll notice that these are mostly from plant sources. You should try and include a few variations of these items into each meal you eat. Olive oil should be the main fat you use in your cooking and your dishes, so replace any other butter or cooking oil you used to use. Generous uses of herbs and spices are also encouraged to season your food and add flavor as an alternative to salt. If you don't have access to fresh herbs, you can buy the dried version. Always be sure to read the nutrition labels to ensure there are no other ingredients mixed with the herbs. Fresh ginger and garlic are also great flavor enhancers for your meals. They can be easily stored in the freezer.

Fish & seafood: These are important staples of the Mediterranean diet that should be consumed often as a protein source. You want to try and include these in your diet at least two times a week. Try new varieties of fish, either frozen or fresh. Also incorporate seafood like mussels, crab, and shrimp into your diet. Canned tuna is also great to include on sandwiches or toss in a salad with fresh vegetables.

Cheese, yogurt, eggs & poultry: These ingredients should be consumed in more moderate amounts when on the Mediterranean diet. Depending on the food, they should be used sparingly throughout the week. Keep in mind that if you are using eggs in baking or cooking, those will also be counted in your weekly limit. You want to stick to more healthy cheese like Parmesan, ricotta, or feta that you can add as a topping or garnish on your dishes.

Red meat & sweets: These items are going to be consumed less frequently when on the Mediterranean diet. If you are eating them, you want to be sure it is only in small quantities and prefer lean meat versions with less fat. Most studies recommend a maximum of 12 to

16 ounces per month. You can still have red meat on occasion to add some variety to your diet, but you want to reduce how often you have it. That's because of all the health concerns that come with sugar and red meat. The Mediterranean diet is working to improve cardiovascular health and reduce blood pressure, while red meat tends to be dangerous in terms of cardiac health. The residents of Greece ate very little red meat and instead had fish or seafood as their main source of protein.

Water: The Mediterranean diet encourages you to be hydrated so that means drinking more than your daily intake of water. The Institute of Medicine recommends a total of 9 cups each day for women, and 13 cups for men. If a woman is pregnant or breastfeeding, that number should be increased.

Wine: Moderate consumption of wine with meals is encouraged on the Mediterranean diet. Studies have shown that moderate consumption of alcohol can reduce the risk of heart disease. That can mean about 1 glass per day for women. Men tend to have higher body mass so they can consume 1 to 2 glasses. Please keep in mind what your doctor would recommend regarding wine consumption based on your individual health and family history.

What To Eat: The Mediterranean Diet Food List

The Mediterranean diet is a very beneficial diet. That said, it is very hard for you to experience any of the benefits that you have just learned without following the diet to the latter. One way of doing that is by eating what the diet allows and avoiding what the diet prohibits you to eat. Let's get started

What you can eat

The foods you can eat while you are on a Mediterranean diet fall into two categories. There are those foods that you can eat regularly and there are those that you should only eat in moderation. Here is an extensive list of both categories.

Foods to eat regularly

Healthy fats like avocado oil, avocados, olives and extra virgin olive oil

Fruits like peaches, figs, melons, dates, bananas, strawberries, grapes, pears, oranges, and apples. Note that you can eat most fruits while on this diet

Vegetables like cucumbers, Brussels sprouts, artichoke, eggplant, carrots, cauliflower, onions, spinach, kale, broccoli and tomatoes. Those are just popular examples but basically all vegetables are allowed in the Mediterranean diet

Whole grains like pasta, whole wheat, whole grain bread, corn, buckwheat, barley, rye, brown rice and whole oats.

Nuts and seeds like pumpkin seeds, cashews, pistachios, walnuts, almonds and macadamia nuts

Herbs and spices; the best herbs and spices are mostly fresh and dried like mint, rosemary, cinnamon, basil and pepper.

Tubers like sweet potatoes, yams, turnips and potatoes.

Legumes like chickpeas, peanuts, pulses, lentils, peas and beans.

Fish and seafood, which are actually your primary source of protein. Good examples include shellfish like crab, mussels and oysters, shrimp, tuna, haddock and salmon.

Foods You Should Eat In Moderation

You should only eat the below foods less frequently when compared to the foods in the list above.

Red meat like bacon, ground beef and steak

Dairy products low in fat or fat free. Some of the popular examples include cheese, yogurt and low fat milk

Eggs, as they are good sources of proteins and are healthier when poached and boiled

Poultry like duck, turkey and chicken

Note that chicken are healthy when their skin is removed. This is because you reduce the cholesterol in the chicken.

Later on in the book, this list of foods that you are allowed to eat when on a Mediterranean diet will be expanded further where you will know what foods to take on a daily, weekly and monthly basis.

Food to Avoid

The below list contains a couple of foods that you need to avoid when on a Mediterranean diet completely. This is because they are unhealthy and when you eat them, you will be unable to experience the benefits of a Mediterranean diet. These foods include;

Processed meat- you should avoid processed meats like bacon, sausage and hot dogs because they are high in saturated fats, which are unhealthy.

Refined oils - stay away from unhealthy oils like cottonseed oil, vegetable oil and soybean oil.

Saturated or Trans-fats - good example of these fats include butter and margarine.

Highly processed foods – avoid all highly processed foods. By this, I mean all the foods that are packaged. This can be packaged crisp, nuts, wheat etc. Some of these foods are marked and labeled low fat but are actually quite high in sugar.

Refined grains - avoid refined grains like refined pasta, white bread, cereals, bagels etc

Added sugar- foods, which contain added sugar like sodas, chocolates, candy and ice cream should be completely avoided. If you have a sweet tooth, you can substitute products with added sugar with natural sweeteners.

Now that you know what to eat and what not to eat when on the Mediterranean diet you are now ready to learn how you can adopt the diet. The next chapter will show you how to do that.

Common Mistakes

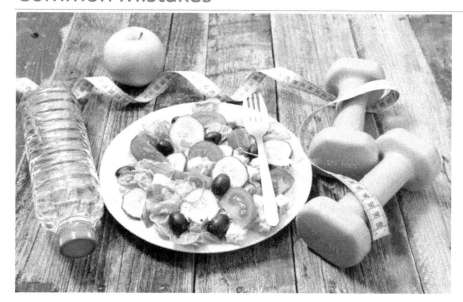

When you start a new diet, you will make some mistakes or encounter situations in which you don't know what to do. Before you get on the Mediterranean diet plan, here is a heads up about common mistakes that people make. If you know about these mistakes, you can avoid them and achieve success more quickly.

- All or nothing

Your attitude towards the diet matters a lot. This is why you must make sure you are mentally prepared for the diet. It will be different from your ordinary lifestyle, which is why you need an abundance of information about it. To learn the benefits of this diet, you can ask the experts or people who have experienced it. You may experience mood or physical changes while adopting this lifestyle but there is nothing to worry about because it is all for your own benefit. When you see this diet as all or nothing you are looking at it from a short-term perspective and will end up abandoning it. Instead, be prepared to follow this diet strictly so that you will see a big difference.

- The same things

Don't eat the same things over and over again, every day. One of the most common mistakes people make is that they think that eating the same kind of vegetables all week long will help them lose weight. This is incorrect. You must have variety in your diet. The Mediterranean diet doesn't require that you consume only one ingredient all week long. It allows you to have multiple kinds of dishes throughout the week, but maintain portion control. You can eat chicken and eggs, but control your portions and eat according to the point system you have established for yourself. By the end of this book, you will be able to create a meal plan that will help you eat different kinds of food all week long. Don't eat the same things all the time because then you will be losing nutrients, which will eventually make you weak.

- Deprivation

Another mistake people make is thinking that deprivation is the only way to lose weight. The main point of this diet plan is to give you energy while helping you lose weight. Deprivation will only make you weaker. This diet plan won't work if you don't eat at all, so be sure to stick this point in your brain.

- Giving up

Don't give up in the middle of the Mediterranean diet because then it will have been of no use. If you see yourself losing weight and you think, 'Now I can have sweet things" … well, that's not the way to do it. If you have decided to follow it, do so. Stick to it no matter what. If you have cravings for chocolate, find a healthy alternative rather than giving up. This way, you will develop self-control and won't get into bad eating habits. Our bodies need time to adjust and stabilize in terms of the food we eat, which is why switching back and forth is never a good option.

- Not setting goals

One of the main mistakes people make is not setting goals when they start the diet. You must have a goal in terms of how much weight you want to lose and work accordingly. Some people may take six months to reach their goal, while some many take only months. It depends on your body type and the goal you set. If you like to go slow, that is your goal and you won't see an immediate difference. On the other hand, if you have a goal to lose five pounds in one month, you will be sticking strictly to the diet plan without missing a meal. When you don't have a plan, you will become distracted and be unable to reach your destination, no matter how hard you try.

- Following the wrong plan

Another common mistake is that you don't have enough knowledge about the plan you are following to lose weight. Maybe you are following the wrong plan, one that doesn't seem to work for you. If you're confused, don't make the decision by yourself to follow the Mediterranean plan; instead, consult an expert who can advise you on what to eat and do to adopt a healthy lifestyle. Many people follow their own style while mixing in elements of the Mediterranean diet, but if you try to modify the dishes, you won't achieve the optimal results. Make sure you follow the plan and prepare the correct recipes at home.

Eating Out On The Mediterranean Diet

It has been scientifically proven that the best and effective diets are mostly the ones that work with the body's natural process and internal environment to bring about the positive changes.

What Should you Have on Your Plate?

By now, you should already have a good idea of what to eat on the Mediterranean diet, but just to summarize:

•   You should try to include fruits, seeds, nuts, vegetables, potatoes, bread, whole grain, herbs, fish, spices, seafood liberally and keep them in your platter.

•   Eggs, yogurt, cheese, and poultry should be eaten in moderation.

•   Beef, pork and other red meats should be eaten rarely or as minimally as possible.

•   Completely avoid processed meat, sugar, sweetened beverages and refined grains from reaching your plate.

Your Shopping Guide

Aside from knowing how to start your diet, you should also know a little bit about how-to set-up your pantry.

What to go for

•   All kinds of vegetables including tomatoes, kale, broccoli, spinach, cauliflower, Brussels sprouts, carrots, cucumbers, etc.

•   All types of fruits such as orange, apple, banana, pears, grapes, dates, strawberries, figs, melons, peaches, etc.

- Nuts and seeds such as almonds, Macadamia, walnuts, cashews, sunflower seeds, pumpkin seeds, etc.

- Legumes such as beans, lentils, peas, pulses, chickpeas etc.

- Tubers such as yams, turnips, potatoes, sweet potatoes and so on

- Whole grains such as whole oats, rye, brown rice, corn, barley, buckwheat, whole wheat, whole grain pasta, and bread

- Fish and seafood such as sardines, salmon, tuna, shrimp, mackerel, oyster, crab, clams, mussels, etc.

- Poultry such as turkey, chicken, duck and more

- Eggs including duck, quail and chicken eggs

- Dairy such as cheese, Greek yogurt, etc.

- Herbs and spices such as mint, basil, garlic, rosemary, cinnamon, sage, pepper, etc.

- Healthy fats and oil such as extra virgin olive oil, avocado oil, olives, etc.

What to avoid

- Foods with added sugar such as soda, ice cream, candies, table sugar, etc.

- Refined grains such as white bread or pasta made with refined wheat

- Margarine and similar processed foods that contain Trans Fats

- Refined oil such as cottonseed oil, soybean oil, etc.

- Processed meat such as hot dogs, processed sausages and so on

- Highly processed food with labels such as "Low-Fat" or "Diet" or anything that is not natural

Oils to know about

The Mediterranean Diet emphasizes healthy oils. The following are some of the oils that you might want to consider.

Coconut Oil: This particular oil is semi-solid at room temperature and can be used for months without it turning rancid.

This particular oil also has a lot of health benefits! Since this oil is rich in a fatty acid known as Lauric Acid, it can help to improve cholesterol levels and kill various pathogens.

Extra-Virgin Olive Oil: Olive Oils are renowned worldwide for being one of the healthiest oils, and this is exactly why the Mediterranean Diet uses this oil as its key ingredient.

Some recent studies have shown that olive oil can even help to improve health biomarkers such as increasing the HDL cholesterol and lowering the amount of bad LDL cholesterol.

Avocado Oil: The composition of Avocado oil is very similar to olive oil and as such, it holds similar health benefits. It can be used for many purposes as an alternative for olive oil (Such as cooking).

Healthy salt alternatives

Asides from replacing healthy oils, the Mediterranean Diet will also ask you to opt for healthy salt alternatives as well. Below are some that you might want to consider.

Sunflower Seeds

Sunflower seeds are excellent and give a nutty and sweet flavor.

Fresh Squeezed Lemon

Lemon is believed to a be a nice hybrid between citron and bitter orange. These are packed with Vitamin C, which helps to neutralize damaging free radicals from the system.

Onion Powder

Onion powder is a dehydrated ground spice made from onion bulb, which is mostly used as a seasoning and is a fine salt alternative.

Black Pepper Powder

The black pepper powder is also a salt alternative that is native to India. Use it by grinding whole peppercorns!

Cinnamon

Cinnamon is very well-known as a savory spice, and two varieties are available: Ceylon and Chinese. Both of them sport a kind of sharp, warm and sweet flavor.

Flavored Vinegar

Fruit infused vinegar or flavored vinegar as we call it in our book are mixtures of vinegar that are combined with fruits in order to give a nice flavor. These are excellent ingredients to add a bit of flavor to meals without salt. Experimentation might be required to find the perfect fruit blend for you.

As for the process of making the vinegar:

- Wash your fruits and slice them well

- Place ½ a cup of your fruit in a mason jar

- Top them up with white wine vinegar (or balsamic vinegar)

- Allow them to sit for 2 weeks or so

- Strain and use as needed

Eating Out on the Mediterranean Diet

Initially, it might seem a little bit confusing, but eating out at a restaurant while on a Mediterranean Diet is actually pretty easy. Just follow the steps below:

• Try to ensure that you choose seafood or fish as the main dish of your meal

• When ordering, try to make a special request and ask the restaurant to fry their food using extra virgin olive oil

• Ask for only whole-grain based ingredients if possible

• If possible, try to read the menu of the restaurant before going there

• Try to have a simple snack before you go to the restaurant; this will help prevent you from overeating

Getting Started with the Mediterranean Diet and Meal Planning

The Mediterranean diet is a straightforward, easy to follow, and delicious diet, but you need a bit of preparation. Preparing for the Mediterranean diet is largely about preparing yourself for a new way of eating and adjusting your attitude toward food into one of joyful expectation and appreciation of good meals and good company.

Planning Your Mediterranean Diet

There are a few things to make your transition to the diet easier and effortless.

Ease your way into more healthful eating:

Before starting the diet, it can be helpful to spend a week or two cutting back on the least healthful foods that you are currently eating. You might start with fast food or eliminate cream-based sauces and soups. You can begin by cutting back on processed foods like frozen meals, boxed dinners, and chips. Some other things to start trimming might be sodas, coffee with a lot of sugar, and milk. You should lower butter, and cut out red meats such as lamb, beef, and pork.

Start thinking about what you'll be eating:

Just like planning for a vacation, you need to plan your diet. Go through the list of foods you need to eat on the Mediterranean diet and get recipe and meal ideas.

Gather what you'll need:

Everything in the Mediterranean diet is easily found at farmers' markets, grocery stores, and seafood shops. Find out where your local farmers' markets are and spend a leisurely morning checking out what is available. Talk to the farmers about what they harvest and when. Building relationships with those vendors can lead to getting special deals and the best selection. You can join the CSA (Community Supported Agriculture) farm nearby. CSA farms are small farms that sell subscription packages of whatever they're growing that season.

For a moderate seasonal or weekly fee, the farm will supply you with enough of that week's harvest to feed your whole family. Freshness is important when following the Mediterranean diet. Joining a CSA is a great way to enjoy the freshness and peak flavor that is so important to the Mediterranean diet. The same is true for your local seafood market and butcher shop. Find out who's selling the freshest, most healthful meats and seafood and buy from them. When you're ready to start, create a shopping list and get as many of your ingredients from your new sources as you can.

Plan your week:

Planning ahead is essential to success. The diet is heavily plant-based, and you need to load up on fresh fruits, vegetables, and herbs each week. By keeping your pantry stocked with whole grains like whole-wheat pasta, polenta, dried or canned beans and legumes, olive oil, and even some canned, vegetables and fish, you can be sure that you'll always have the ingredients for a healthy meal.

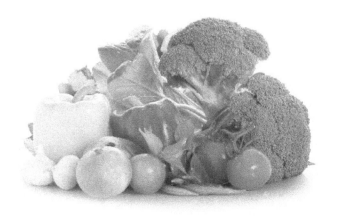

Adjust your portions:

The idea behind the Mediterranean diet is to make up the bulk of your diet with plant-based foods like fruits, vegetables, whole grains, beans, and nuts. Foods like cheese, meat, and sweets are allowed, but they are consumed only occasionally and in small portions. One way to ensure that you're eating enough plant-based foods while following the Mediterranean diet is to fill half your plate with vegetables and fruit, then fill one-quarter with whole grains, and the last quarter your plate with protein such as beans, fish, shellfish, or poultry. Once every week or two, enjoy a small serving of red meat, such as beef or lamb, or use meat as an accent to add flavor to plant-based stews, sauces, or other dishes. Here are some guidelines that will help you visualize appropriate portions for the Mediterranean diet:

- One ½ cup serving of grains or beans are about the size of the palm of your hand.
- 1 cup of vegetables is as big as a baseball.
- One medium piece of fruit is as big as a tennis ball.
- One 1-ounce serving of cheese is about the size of a pair of dice.
- One 3-ounce portion of meat (pork, lamb, fish, beef, or poultry) is roughly the size of a deck of cards.

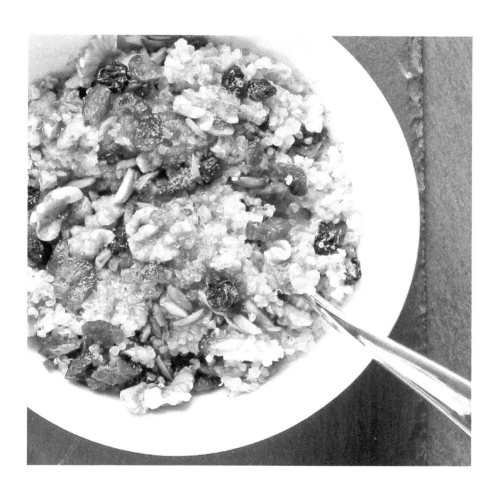

Caprese Poached Eggs

Preparation Time: 10 minutes

Cooking Time: 10 minutes

Servings: 2

Ingredients:

- 1 tablespoon white vinegar (distilled)
- 4 eggs
- 1 tomato (sliced)
- 2 mozzarella cheese slices (1 ounce each)
- 4 teaspoon pesto
- 2 whole wheat English muffins
- 2 teaspoons sea salt.

Directions:

Place a large saucepan on your stove and fill it with 3 inches of water. Turn the heat to high so that the water can come to a boil. When the water starts boiling, add the tablespoon of vinegar to the saucepan and the salt, reduce the heat so that the water will maintain a gentle boil.

As the water simmers, Prepare your English muffins. Cut the muffins in half lengthwise. Place a slice of the mozzarella cheese on each muffin half then layer on a slice of tomato. Place the muffins on a cooking sheet and place them in your boiler. If you have a toaster oven you can use that instead of your broiler. Allow the muffins to toast up and the cheese to soften. This should take about 5 minutes.

As the muffins toast, crack an egg into a small bowl. Hold the bowl over the saucepan with the simmering water. Slowly pour the egg into the water, being careful not to break the yolk. Then repeat with the other three eggs. Once all eggs are in the water allow them to poach for about 3 minutes. The egg whites should be firm and fluffy.

As the eggs cook, place a few paper towels on a plate. Use a slotted spoon to transfer your cooked eggs to the plate to remove any excess water.

Remove your English muffin from the boiler or toaster oven.

Carefully transfer the muffin halves to a serving plate and place a poached egg on each half.

Take your pesto sauce and top each muffin with a tablespoon of the sauce. Serve and enjoy!

Nutrition:

Calories: 357

Carbs: 19 g

Protein: 23 g

Fat: 21.5 g

Sautéed Greens and Eggs

Preparation Time: 15 minutes

Cooking Time: 15 minutes

Servings: 4

Ingredients:

- 1 tablespoon virgin olive oil
- 4 eggs
- 2 cups rainbow chard
- 1 cup spinach
- ½ cup arugula
- 2 garlic cloves (minced)
- ½ cup feta cheese
- ½ teaspoon sea salt
- ½ teaspoon black pepper

Directions:

Place a large skillet on your stove with the tablespoon of virgin olive oil. Turn the heat on to medium-high.

As the skillet is heating, break your eggs into a medium-sized mixing bowl and use a fork to beat the eggs. Set to the side.

Your skillet should be nice and hot now. Add in your rainbow chard, spinach, and arugula and allow the greens to sauté for about 5 minutes. Once the greens are nice and tender, add your minced garlic to the skillet and cook for two minutes.

Take your egg mixture and pour it into the skillet with your greens. Then sprinkle your feta cheese over top.

Cover the pan and then allow it to cook for 6 minutes.

Once the eggs have cooked thoroughly, uncover the skillet and sprinkle the sea salt and black pepper over top.

Divide the mixture into four and serve!

Nutrition:

Calories: 152

Protein: 9.2 G

Fat: 11.9 G

Carbs: 3 G

Breakfast Pizza

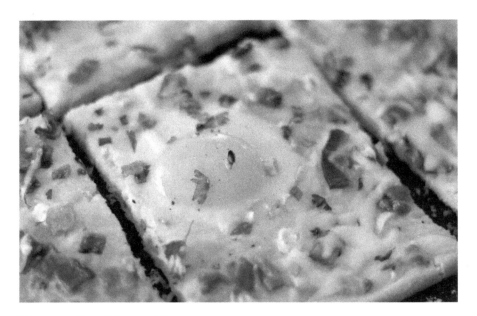

Preparation Time: 15 minutes

Cooking Time: 20 minutes

Servings: 4

Ingredients:

- 2 tablespoons virgin olive oil
- 4 eggs
- ¼ onion (chopped)
- ½ tomato (diced)
- ½ cup spinach (chopped)
- ½ cup mushroom (chopped)
- 1 avocado (pit and peel removed, sliced)
- 2 tablespoons pesto
- 2 pita bread
- ½ cup mozzarella cheese (shredded)

Directions:

Start by lining a cookie sheet with a parchment paper and set it to the side.

Start getting your oven nice and hot by preheating it to 350 degrees F.

Take a large skillet and place it on top of your stove. Pour in 1 tablespoon of the virgin olive oil. Turn the heat to medium-high. Add the chopped onions to your skillet and let them cook for 5 minutes. The onions should be translucent. Transfer the onions in a small bowl and then set it aside.

Add the remaining 1 tablespoon of olive oil to the skillet.

In a bowl, crack the eggs and then gently beat it together with a fork. Pour the mixture into the skillet. Cook the eggs for about 5 minutes, stir occasionally so that they cook evenly. Turn off the heat when they are cooked completely.

Take your Prepared cookie sheet and place the pita bread on it. Spread a tablespoon of your pesto on each pita. Top each pita with half the spinach, eggs, onions, tomatoes, mushrooms, and mozzarella cheese.

Place the cookie sheet into the oven for 10 minutes.

Remove the cookie sheet from the oven, then lay the sliced avocado over the top and enjoy!

Nutrition:

Calories: 361

Protein: 12 G

Fat: 26 G

Carbs: 24.3 G

Caprese on Sourdough

Preparation Time: 10 minutes

Cooking Time: 10 minutes

Servings: 4

Ingredients:

- 1 tablespoon extra-virgin olive oil
- 1 garlic clove (peeled)
- 1 tomato (sliced)
- 4 thick slices of mozzarella cheese
- 8 basil leaves (fresh)
- 1 teaspoon oregano
- 1 tablespoon balsamic vinegar
- 4 slices of sourdough bread

Directions:

Begin by toasting your sourdough bread. This is easiest to do if you have a toaster oven, but you can also place it on a baking sheet and then place them under your broiler for a minute or two, flip them so that each side is toasted.

Once your sourdough is nicely toasted take your peeled garlic clove and rub one side of each slice of bread.

Place two basil leaves on each piece of sourdough and a slice or two of tomatoes. Top with a thick slice of mozzarella cheese.

Drizzle a little bit of the olive oil and balsamic vinegar over top. Finish each slice with a sprinkle of oregano.

Nutrition:

Calories: 196

Protein: 11.3 G

Fat: 9 G

Carbs: 17.2 G

Mediterranean Inspired Breakfast Quinoa

Preparation Time: 20 minutes

Cooking Time: 35 minutes

Servings: 4

Ingredients:

- 1 cup quinoa (cooked)
- 2 cups low-fat milk
- 3 Medjool dates (pitted, chopped fine)
- 1 apple (cored, chopped)
- ¼ cup almonds (chopped)
- 1 teaspoon pure vanilla extract
- 1 teaspoon cinnamon (ground)
- 2 tablespoon honey (optional)

Directions:

Place a medium-sized skillet on your stove. Add in your chopped almonds, turn the heat to medium, and allow them to toast for about 5 minutes. When they are a nice golden brown turn the heat off and set them to the side.

Next, take a medium-sized saucepan and place it on your stove. Turn up the heat just a bit to medium-high. Add in your quinoa and cinnamon and warm for 3 minutes. Then pour in the milk and add your chopped apple. Wait for it to boil. Once at a steady boil, cover the saucepan and reduce the heat to medium-low. Let all the flavors simmer for 20 minutes. Then add in the vanilla, dates, and half the toasted almost. Stir everything and cook for another 2 minutes.

Remove the from the heat and divide into four equal portions. Top with the remaining almonds and drizzle honey over top if you like it to be a little sweeter.

Nutrition:

Calories: 225

Protein: 81 G

Fat: 53 G

Carbs: 37.2 G

Eggs Florentine

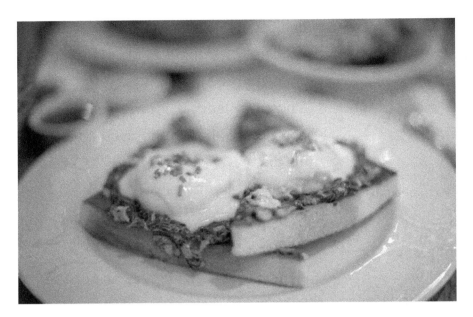

Preparation Time: 15 minutes

Cooking Time: 20 minutes

Servings: 4

Ingredients:

- 1 tablespoon virgin olive oil
- 6 eggs
- 2 garlic cloves (minced)
- ½ onion (finely diced)
- ½ cup mushrooms (sliced)
- 2 cups spinach (chopped)
- 2 tomatoes (diced)
- 1 teaspoon oregano (dried)
- 1 teaspoon basil (dried)
- ¼ cup feta (crumbles)

- ¼ teaspoon black pepper

Directions:

Place a large skillet on your stove with the virgin olive oil in it. Turn the heat to medium. Add the garlic and diced onions to the skillet. Let the flavors of the onion and garlic cook together for 2 minutes then add the mushroom and spinach and cook for another 5 minutes.

As the spinach and mushrooms cook, crack your eggs into a small mixing bowl and lightly beat them with a fork. Once the spinach has droop, pour the egg mixture into the skillet. Sprinkle on the oregano, basil, and black pepper. Cover the pan and then let the eggs get cooked for about 3 to 5 minutes, just until they are firm enough to flip.

Once you have flipped your eggs sprinkle the crumbled feta and tomatoes on top and cook for another 5 minutes.

Once everything has cooked thoroughly turn off the heat and cut into 4 equal portions and enjoy.

Nutrition:

Calories: 174

Protein: 11.2 G

Fat: 12.3 G

Carbs: 6.1 G

Egg White Breakfast Sandwich

Preparation Time: 5 minutes

Cooking Time: 10 minutes

Servings: 2

Ingredients:

- 1 tablespoon virgin olive oil
- 4 egg whites
- ½ cup spinach
- 1 tomato (sliced)
- 2 whole-grain English muffins

Directions:

Place a medium-sized skillet on your stove and turn the heat to medium. Pour in the virgin olive oil to warm.

Lightly beat your egg whites in a small mixing bowl and then pour into your skillet. Allow the egg whites to cook for about 3 minutes, flip and cook for 3 more minutes on the other side. When fully cooked, the whites should be firm and fluffy. Turn off the heat.

Slice your English muffins in half and place them in your toaster oven. Remove once toasted.

Divide your cooked egg whites into two equal portions and place on one slice of your toasted English muffin. Layer on your sliced tomatoes and spinach. Place the other half of your English muffin on top and enjoy!

Nutrition:

Calories: 261

Protein: 14.6 G

Fat: 9.2 G

Carbs: 31.8G

Mediterranean Egg Wrap

Preparation Time: 5 minutes

Cooking Time: 10 minutes

Servings: 2

Ingredients:

- 1 tablespoon virgin olive oil
- 4 eggs
- 2 cups spinach (chopped)
- 2 sundried tomatoes (chopped)
- 2 tomatoes (diced)
- ½ cup feta cheese (crumbled)
- 2 whole-wheat tortillas

Directions:

Begin by placing a large skillet on your stove. Pour in the virgin olive oil and turn up the heat to medium-high. Crack your eggs in a small mixing bowl while waiting for the oil to be hot and then use a fork to beat the eggs together lightly. Set the eggs to the side.

Once the oil in the skillet has been heating up for a few minutes add in your spinach and sundried tomatoes. Allow the spinach to cook for about 3 minutes or until it begins to wilt. Then pour in the eggs. Use a spatula to scramble the mixture as it cooks. Let the eggs cook for about 3 minutes. Sprinkle the feta cheese and then cook for another minute. Turn the heat all the way off.

Heat up your tortillas for 30 seconds in your microwave. Then divide your egg mixture between the two tortillas. Top each with diced tomatoes.

Fold in two sides of your tortilla and then roll like a burrito.

You can place it in a warm skillet so that the wrap holds its shape better or you can just enjoy it as is!

Nutrition:

Calories: 371

Protein: 20 G

Fat: 24.8 G

Carbs: 19.9 G

Quinoa Bowl

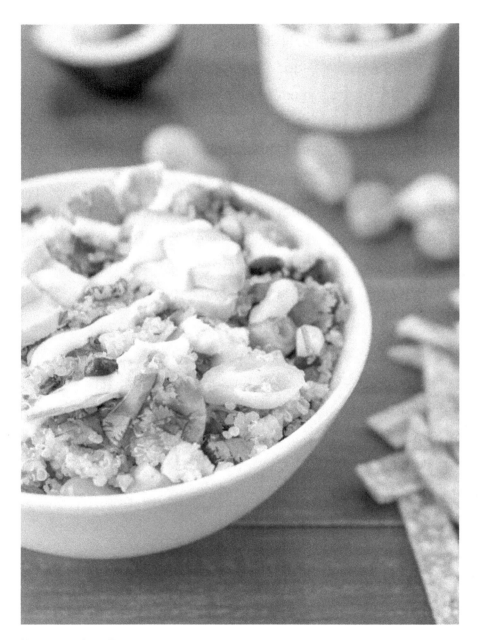

Preparation Time: 10 minutes

Cooking Time: 15 minutes

Servings: 6

Ingredients:

- 2 c. quinoa
- 1 c. blueberries
- 1 c. unsweetened coconut milk
- 2 c. water
- 2 tbsps. almonds
- 1 tsp. pistachio
- 2 tbsps. honey

Directions:

Combine the coconut milk and water in the saucepan and stir the liquid well.

Add the quinoa and close the lid.

Cook the mixture on medium heat for 5 minutes.

Wash the blueberries carefully and add them to the quinoa mixture.

Stir it carefully and continue to cook for 2 minutes. At the same time Combine the pistachio and almonds and crush the nuts.

Sprinkle the quinoa with the crushed nuts and cook the mixture for 3 minutes more.

Add honey and stir the mixture carefully for about 5 minutes until the honey has dissolved.

Transfer to serving bowls and enjoy.

Nutrition:

Calories: 348

Protein: 9.6 G

Fat: 14.1 G

Carbs: 48.3 G

Yogurt Figs Mix

Preparation Time: 10 minutes

Cooking Time: 10 minutes

Servings: 4

Ingredients:

- 8 oz. or 227 g chopped figs
- 2 c. Greek yogurt
- 1 tbsp. honey
- 1 tsp. cinnamon powder
- 1 tbsp. chopped almonds
- 1 tbsp. chopped walnuts
- ¼ c. pistachios, chopped

Directions:

Adjust your heat to medium. Set a pan in place and stir in the ingredients apart from yogurt. Cook for about 5 minutes.

Divide yogurt in serving bowls. Top with figs mixture and toss gently.

Serve and enjoy.

Nutrition:

Calories: 198

Protein: 3.4 G

Fat: 4.2 G

Carbs: 42.1 G

Seeds and Lentils Oats

Preparation Time: 10 minutes

Cooking Time: 50 minutes

Servings: 4

Ingredients:

- ½ c. red lentils
- ¼ c. toasted pumpkin seeds
- 2 tsps. olive oil
- ¼ c. rolled oats
- ¼ c. shredded coconut flesh,
- 1 tbsps. honey
- 1 tbsp. orange zest, grated
- 1 c. Greek yogurt
- 1 c. blackberries

Directions:

Preheat your oven to 370 F/187 C.

Line a parchment paper on your baking sheet and grease with olive oil. Set the lentils and place them in the oven, and roast for about 30 minutes.

Toss in the remaining ingredients with exception of berries and yogurt. Continue to bake for 20 more minutes.

Set in a bowl and toss in berries and yogurt. Divide in serving plates and enjoy.

Nutrition:

Calories: 204

Protein: 9.5 G

Fat: 7.1 G

Carbs: 27.6 G

Cinnamon Apple and Lentils Porridge

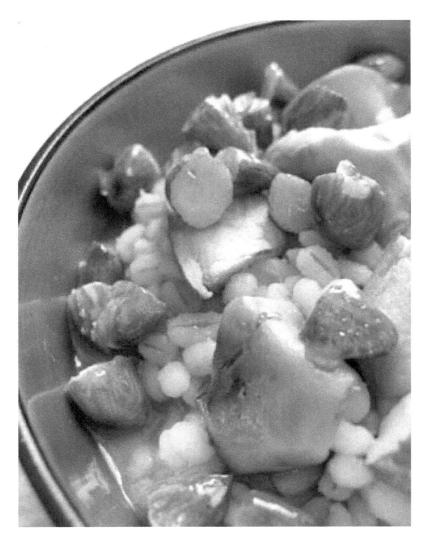

Preparation Time: 5 minutes

Cooking Time: 10 minutes

Servings: 4

Ingredients:

- ½ c. chopped walnuts
- 2 cored green apples, peeled and cubed

- 3 tbsps. maple syrup
- 3 c. almond milk
- ½ c. red lentils
- ½ tsp. cinnamon powder
- ½ c. dried cranberries
- 1 tsp. vanilla extract

Directions:

Set your heat to medium and set a pot in place. Add in milk to heat for a minute. Toss in the remaining ingredients.

Simmer for approximately 12 minutes.

Set in serving plates and enjoy.

Nutrition:

Calories: 150

Protein: 5 G

Fat: 2 G

Carbs: 3 G

Coriander Mushroom Salad

Preparation Time: 10 minutes

Cooking Time: 1 minutes

Servings: 6

Ingredients:

- ½ lb. or 220 g sliced white mushrooms
- 1 tbsp. olive oil
- 3 minced garlic cloves
- Salt and black pepper
- 1 diced tomato
- 1 pitted avocado, peeled and cubed
- 3 tbsps. lime juice
- ½ c. chicken stock or water
- 2 tbsps. chopped coriander

Directions:

Adjust your heat to medium. Using a pan, heat your olive oil and add in mushrooms to sauté for about 5 minutes.

Put all the rest of the ingredients and cook for 7 more minutes.

Serve and enjoy.

Nutrition:

Calories: 159.2

Protein: 5.2 G

Fat: 15 G

Carbs: 3.4 G

Feta Baked Eggs

Preparation Time: 5 minutes

Cooking Time: 15 minutes

Servings: 2

Ingredients:

- 1 tsp. butter
- ½ tsp. olive oil
- 2 eggs
- ¼ tsp. onion powder
- ¼ tsp. chili flakes
- 2 oz. or 57 g Feta cheese
- 1 tsp. freshly chopped dill

Directions:

Toss butter in the skillet.

Add olive oil and bring it to boil.

After this, crack the eggs in the skillet.

Sprinkle them with chili flakes and onion powder.

Then preheat the oven to 360°F

Transfer the skillet with eggs in the oven and cook for 10 minutes. Then crumble Feta cheese and sprinkle it over the eggs.

Bake the eggs for 5 minutes more

Top with chopped dill and serve.

Nutrition:

Calories: 167

Protein: 9.7 G

Fat: 13.5 G

Carbs: 2 G

Banana Oats

Preparation Time: 10 minutes

Cooking Time: 0 minutes

Servings: 2

Ingredients:

- ½ cup cold brewed coffee

- 2 dates, pitted

- 2 tablespoons cocoa powder

- 1 cup rolled oats

- 1 and ½ tablespoons chia seeds

Directions:

1. In a blender, combine the 1 banana with the ¾ almond milk and the rest of the ingredients, pulse, divide into bowls and serve for breakfast.

Nutrition:

451 calories

25g fat

9.9g fiber

Berry Oats

Preparation Time: 5 minutes

Cooking Time: 0 minute

Servings: 2

Ingredients:

- ½ cup rolled oats
- 1 cup almond milk
- ¼ cup chia seeds
- 2 teaspoons honey
- 1 cup berries, pureed

Directions:

1. In a bowl, combine the oats with the milk and the rest of the ingredients except 1 tbsp. of yogurt, toss, divide into bowls, top with the yogurt and serve cold for breakfast.

Nutrition:

420 calories

30g fat

6.4g protein

Muesli and Fresh Fruits Oatmeal

Preparation Time: 10 minutes

Cooking Time: 0 minutes

Servings: 4

Ingredients:

- 3 cups water
- 1 cup almond milk
- 1 tablespoon sugar
- 2 cups oatmeal
- 1 cups Muesli
- Fresh fruits as you prefer

Directions:

1. In a pan, scourge water with the milk, bring to a boil over medium heat.
2. The cook the oats about 10 minutes
3. Add sugar and stir the oats and cook for 5 minutes.
4. Divide the mix into bowls, sprinkle with muesli and fresh fruits and serve for breakfast.

Nutrition:

170 calories

17.8g fat

1.5g protein

Quinoa Muffins

Preparation Time: 10 minutes

Cooking Time: 30 minutes

Servings: 12

Ingredients:

- 6 eggs, whisked
- 1 cup Swiss cheese, grated
- 1 small yellow onion, chopped
- 1 cup quinoa, white mushrooms
- ½ cup sun-dried tomatoes, chopped

Directions:

1. In a bowl, combine the eggs with salt, pepper and the rest of the ingredients and whisk well.

2. Divide this into a silicone muffin pan, bake at 350 degrees F for 30 minutes and serve for breakfast.

Nutrition:

123 calories

5.6g fat

7.5g protein

Greek Cheesy Yogurt

Preparation Time: 2 hours in freezer

Cooking Time: 0 minutes

Servings: 4

Ingredients:

- 1 cup Greek yogurt

- 1 tablespoon honey

- ½ cup feta cheese, crumbled

Directions:

1. In a blender, combine the yogurt with the honey and the cheese and pulse well.

2. Divide into bowls and freeze for 2 hours

3. Serve for breakfast.

Nutrition:

161 calories

10g fat

6.6g protein

Walnuts Yogurt Mix

Preparation Time: 10 minutes

Cooking Time: 0 minutes

Servings: 6

Ingredients:

- 2 and ½ cups Greek yogurt
- 1 and ½ cups walnuts, chopped
- 1 teaspoon vanilla extract
- ¾ cup honey
- 2 teaspoons cinnamon powder

Directions:

1. In a bowl, incorporate yogurt with the walnuts and the rest of the ingredients, toss, divide into smaller bowls and keep in the fridge for 10 minutes before serving for breakfast.

Nutrition:

388 calories

24.6g fat

10.2g protein

Tahini Pine Nuts Toast

Preparation Time: 5 minutes

Cooking Time: 0 minute

Servings: 2

Ingredients:

- 2 whole wheat bread slices, toasted

- 1 tablespoon tahini paste

- 2 teaspoons feta cheese, crumbled

- Juice of ½ lemon

- 2 teaspoons pine nuts

Directions:

1. Whisk tahini with the 1 tsp. of water and the lemon juice well and spread over the toasted bread slices.

2. Top each serving with the remaining ingredients and serve for breakfast.

Nutrition:

142 calories

7.6g fat

5.8g protein

Raspberries and Yogurt Smoothie

Preparation Time: 5 minutes

Cooking Time: 0 minutes

Servings: 2

Ingredients:

- 2 cups raspberries

- ½ cup Greek yogurt

- ½ cup almond milk

- ½ teaspoon vanilla extract

Directions:

1. In your blender, combine the raspberries with the milk, vanilla and the yogurt, pulse well, divide into 2 glasses and serve for breakfast.

Nutrition:

245 calories

9.5g fat

1.6g protein

Cottage Cheese and Berries Omelet

Preparation Time: 5 minutes

Cooking Time: 4 minutes

Servings: 1

Ingredients:

- 1 egg, whisked

- 1 teaspoon cinnamon powder

- 1 tablespoon almond milk

- 3 ounces cottage cheese

- 4 ounces blueberries

Directions:

1. Scourge egg with the rest of the ingredients except the oil and toss.

2. Preheat pan with the oil over medium heat, add the eggs mix, spread, cook for 4 minutes on both sides, then serve.

Nutrition:

190 calories

8g fat

2g protein

Banana Cinnamon Fritters

Preparation Time: 15 minutes

Cooking Time: 6 minutes

Serving: 4

Ingredients:

- 1 cup self-rising flour

- 1 egg, beaten

- 3/4 cup sparkling water

- 2 tsp ground cinnamon

- 2-3 bananas, cut diagonally into 4 pieces each

Directions:

1. Sift flour and cinnamon into a bowl and make a well in the center. Add egg and enough sparkling water to mix to a smooth batter.

2. Heat sunflower oil in a saucepan, enough to cover the base by 1-2 inch, so when a tiny batter dropped into the oil sizzles and rises to the surface. Dip banana pieces into the batter, and then fry for 2-3 minutes or until golden. Pull out using slotted spoon and strain on paper towels. Sprinkle with sugar and serve hot.

Nutrition:

209 calories

10g fat

2g protein

French Toast

Preparation Time: 5 min

Cooking Time: 15 min

Servings: 1

Ingredients:

- 1 egg
- 5 ml coconut milk
- 1 tbsp sugar (facoltative)
- 1 pinch of cacao
- 2 slices of bread
- 2 slices of Ham
- 2 slices of Cheese

Directions:

Beat the egg in a skid;

Add all the ingredients as you go. Dip slices of your chosen bread cut similar to pan carrè and cook in a non-stick pan. Stuff with slices of ham and cheese.

Nutrition:

277 Kcal

Chocolat Quinoa Porridge

Preparation Time: 1 min

Cooking Time: 15 min

Servings: 2

Ingredients:

- 5 tbsp quinoa
- 200 ml coconut milk
- 100 ml of water
- 2 tbsp sugar (if you want)
- 2 dark chocolate cubes
- 2 tbsp dark chocolate

Directions:

Put the quinoa, milk, and chosen sweetener in a small saucepan and bring to a boil over medium heat. Stir occasionally and allow to cook for about 10-15 minutes, until the quinoa is soft, translucent and has absorbed all the liquid. If you prefer a creamier consistency add more milk (or water) and cook longer. For a thicker consistency you can add a tablespoon of low-fat yogurt. Pour into a small plate or cup and garnish with fresh or dried fruit, and finally sprinkle to taste with cinnamon or other flavorings and serve.

Greedy Rice Milk

Preparation Time:

Cooking Time:

Servings: 1

Ingredients:

- 1 cup coconut milk
- ¼ cup of rice
- 1 tbsp of sugar
- Vanilla extract
- 1 tbsp dark chocolate
- ½ cup of water.

Directions:

Heat the milk in a saucepan, then pour in the rice just before the milk comes to a boil and cook over low heat, stirring constantly. While cooking, add the vanilla extract or the vanilla bean and, if desired, the sweetener of your choice. Wait for the rice to absorb all the milk and then transfer it on a plate or in a bowl or glass and sprinkle with cinnamon or cocoa powder. For those who love the strong and bitter taste of pure cocoa, you can prepare a homemade cocoa cream as a topping: I use 10 g of bitter cocoa powder and about 30 ml of water and stevia as a sweetener (again, the type of sweetener and the amount depends on personal taste). Enjoy!

Pasta

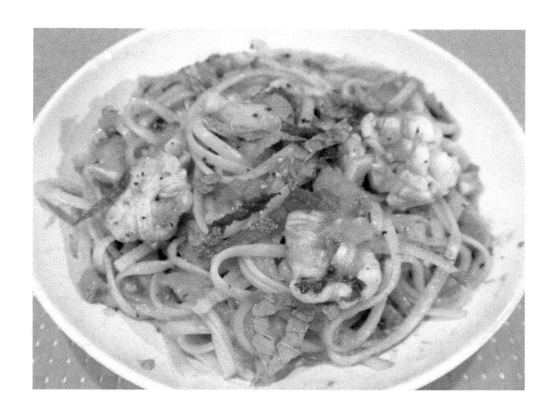

Mediterranean Diet White Bean & Tomato Pasta

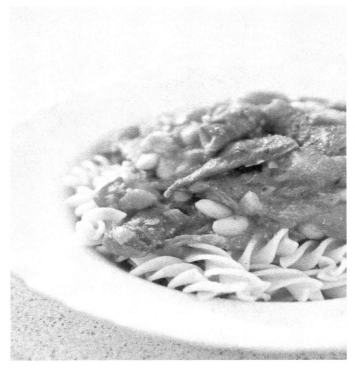

Preparation Time: 10 minutes

Cooking Time: 20 minutes

Servings: 4

Ingredients:

- 2 x 14 & 1/2-oz. cans of diced tomatoes, Italian-style
- 1 x 19-oz. can of drained, rinsed cannellini beans
- 10 oz. of washed, chopped spinach, fresh
- 8 oz. of pasta, penne
- 1/2 cup of feta cheese crumbles

Directions:

Cook pasta using instructions on package. Set aside.

Combine the beans and tomatoes in large-sized, non-stick skillet. Bring to boil on med-high. Then lower heat and allow to simmer for 8-10 minutes.

Add the spinach to sauce. Cook for a couple minutes while constantly stirring, till the spinach has wilted.

Pour sauce over pasta. Sprinkle using feta cheese and serve.

Nutrition:

Calories: 464

Fat: 6.3g

Protein: 22.1g

Carbs: 77g

Shrimp Scampi

Preparation Time: 10 minutes

Cooking Time: 15 minutes

Servings: 4

Ingredients:

- 2 tablespoons extra-virgin olive oil
- 1 shallot, minced
- 1-pound medium shrimp, peeled, deveined, and tails removed
- 6 garlic cloves, minced
- Juice of 1 lemon
- Zest of 1 lemon
- ½ cup dry white wine
- ½ teaspoon sea salt
- ¼ teaspoon freshly ground black pepper
- Pinch red pepper flakes
- ¼ cup chopped fresh Italian parsley leaves
- 6 ounces whole-wheat pasta, cooked according to package directions

Directions:

In a large skillet over medium-high heat, heat the olive oil until it shimmers.

Add the shallot. Cook for about 5 minutes, stir it occasionally, until soft.

Toss in the shrimp. Cook for 3 to 4 minutes, stirring occasionally, until the shrimp is pink.

Add the garlic and cook more for about 30 seconds, stirring constantly.

Stir in the lemon juice and zest, wine, sea salt, pepper, and red pepper flakes. Bring to simmer and then reduce the heat to medium-low. Cook for about 2 minutes until the liquid reduces by half. Remove from the fire and then stir in the parsley.

Toss with the hot pasta and serve.

Nutrition:

Calories: 394

Carbohydrates: 38g

Protein: 32g

Fat: 10g

Lighter Lasagna

Preparation Time: 20 minutes

Cooking Time: 1 hour

Servings: 6

Ingredients:

- 2 Tbsp. olive oil
- 1 onion, finely chopped
- 4 garlic cloves, finely chopped
- 1 ½ lbs. ground beef
- ⅓ Cup red wine
- 2 cups canned chopped tomatoes
- 1 tsp. dried chili flakes
- 1 tsp. each dried oregano, thyme, and rosemary
- Salt and pepper
- 12 sheets (12 halves or 6 whole sheets) fresh lasagna (enough to create three layers across the entire dish)
- Large handful of fresh basil
- 5 oz. fresh Mozzarella, torn

Directions:

Add the olive oil to a large sauté pan over a medium-high heat

Add the onion and garlic to the pan and stir as they soften for about 2 minutes

Add the beef and stir as it turns from pink to brown

Add the red wine and allow the alcohol to burn off for about 2 minutes

Add the tomatoes, chili flakes, herbs, salt and pepper and stir to combine

Leave to simmer for about 30 minutes until thick and rich in flavor

Preheat the oven to 400 degrees Fahrenheit and have a lasagna dish waiting by

Layer the lasagna in this fashion: start with a layer of beef mixture on the bottom, then a layer of pasta, then a few torn basil leaves, repeat until everything has been used, and the top layer is beef sauce (it's not meant to be super tidy, just throw it all together as you please, as long as it's roughly even!)

Finish with the torn Mozzarella and a few extra basil leaves

Bake in the oven for about 30 minutes or until everything is golden and bubbling

Nutrition:

Calories: *714*

Fat: 34 grams

Protein: 50.5 grams

Total carbs: *47.1 grams*

Net carbs: *41 grams*

Greek Pasta Salad

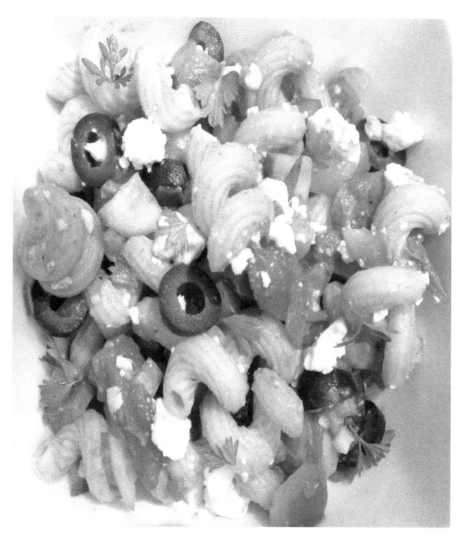

Preparation time: 5 minutes

Cooking time: 11 minutes

Servings: 4

Ingredients:

- Penne pasta (1 cup)

- Lemon juice (1.5 tsp.)

- Red wine vinegar (2 tbsp.)

- Garlic (1 clove)

- Dried oregano (1 tsp.)

- Black pepper and sea salt (as desired)

- Olive oil (.33 cup)

- Halved cherry tomatoes (5)

- Red onion (half of 1 small)

- Green & red bell pepper (half of 1 - each)

- Cucumber (¼ of 1)

- Black olives (.25 cup)

- Crumbled feta cheese (.25 cup)

Directions:

1. Slice the cucumber and olives. Chop/dice the onion, peppers, and garlic. Slice the tomatoes into halves.

2. Arrange a large pot with water and salt using the high-temperature setting. Once it's boiling, add the pasta and cook with the lid off until it's al dente (11 min.). Rinse it using cold water and drain in a colander.

3. Whisk the oil, juice, salt, pepper, vinegar, oregano, and garlic. Combine the cucumber, cheese, olives, peppers, pasta, onions, and tomatoes in a large salad dish.

4. Add the vinaigrette over the pasta and toss. Chill in the fridge (covered) for about three hours and serve as desired.

Nutrition:

Calories: 307

Fats: 23.6 g

Carbs: 19.3 g

Fiber: 2.1 g

Protein: 5.4 g

Insalata Caprese II Salad

Preparation time: 10 minutes

Cooking time: 0 minutes

Servings: 8

Ingredients:

- Orzo pasta (16 oz. pkg.)
- Cooked shrimp (.75 lb.)
- Water-packed artichoke hearts (14 oz. can)
- Sweet red pepper (1 cup)
- Red onion (.75 cup)
- Green pepper (1 cup)
- Pitted Greek olives (.5 cup)
- Parsley (.5 cup)
- Chopped dill (.33 cup)
- Greek vinaigrette (.75 cup)

Directions:

1. Peel and devein the shrimp and cook. Slice each one into thirds (31 to 40 count). Finely chop the onions and peppers.

2. Prepare the orzo, drain, and rinse the orzo with cold water. Drain well. Mince/chop the parsley and dill. Combine the shrimp, orzo, olives, herbs, and veggies.

3. Sprinkle with vinaigrette and toss. Refrigerate and cover until it's time to eat. Serve as a delicious side salad.

Nutrition:

Calories: 397

Fats: 12 g

Carbohydrates: 52 g

Fiber: 3 g

Protein: 18 g

Chopped Israeli Mediterranean Pasta Salad

Preparation time: 15 minutes

Cooking time: 2 minutes

Servings: 8

Ingredients:

- Small bow tie or other small pasta (.5 lb.)

.33 cup of each below:

- Cucumber

- Radish

- Tomato (drain excess liquid)

- Yellow bell pepper

- Orange bell pepper

- Black olives

- Green olives

- Red onions

- Pepperoncini

- Feta cheese

- Fresh thyme leaves

- Dried oregano (1 tsp.)

- Black pepper and salt (as desired)

The Dressing:

Protein: 0.8 g

- 0.25 cup + more, olive oil

- juice of 1 lemon

Directions:

1. Slice the green olives into halves. Dice the feta and pepperoncini. Finely dice the remainder of the veggies.

2. Prepare a pot of water with the salt, and simmer the pasta until it's al dente (checking at two minutes under the listed time). Rinse and drain in cold water.

3. Combine a small amount of oil with the pasta. Add the salt, pepper, oregano, thyme, and veggies. Pour in the rest of the oil, lemon juice, mix and fold in the grated feta.

4. Pop it into the fridge within two hours, best if overnight. Taste test and adjust the seasonings to your liking; add fresh thyme.

Nutrition:

Calories: 65.2

Fats: 5.6 g

Carbohydrates: 4.4 g

Fiber: 1 g

Seafood Linguine

Preparation Time: 45 minutes

Cooking Time: 20 minutes

Servings: 8

Ingredients:

- 1 packet of linguine pasta
- ½ cup chopped red onion
- 3 teaspoons garlic powder
- 1/4 cup olive oil
- 3 cups milk
- 2 teaspoons chopped fresh parsley
- 1/2 cup chopped green pepper
- 1/2 cup chopped red pepper
- 1/2 cup broccoli florets
- 1/2 cup sliced carrots
- 1 cup chopped fresh mushrooms
- 1 cup canned shrimp
- 1 cup crabmeat, drained
- 1 pound scallops

Directions:

Bring a large pot of lightly salted water to a boil. Add linguini and cook for 6 to 8 minutes, or until al dente. Drain.

Meanwhile, fry the red onion and garlic in olive oil in an electric frying pan or large frying pan. Add the milk when the onion is transparent. Boil until bubbles form on the edges of the pan. Add parsley, green and chopped red pepper, broccoli, carrots, mushrooms, shrimps, crab, and scallops and stir until well absorbed.

Remove 1/2 cup of milk from the mixture and place it in a small bowl with the flour. Stir until smooth. Return to the pan with seafood and vegetables. Let the mixture thicken. Season with salt and pepper.

Pour the fish sauce over the cooked and drained linguini noodles. Serve hot.

Nutrition:

418 calories

11 g of fat

52 grams of carbohydrates

28.2 g of protein

69 mg of cholesterol

242 mg of sodium.

Spaghetti Squash with Shrimp Scampi

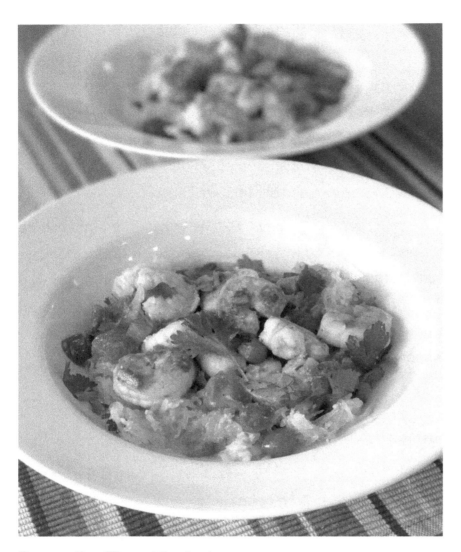

Preparation Time: 30 minutes

Cooking Time: 30 minutes

Servings: 4

Ingredients:

- 2 c. chicken broth
- 1 small onion, chopped

- 2 ½ tsp. lemon-garlic seasoning
- 1 tbsp. butter or ghee
- 3 pounds spaghetti squash, cut crosswise and seeds removed
- ¾ pounds shrimp, shelled and deveined
- Pepper and salt to taste.

Directions:

Pour broth in the Crockpot and stir in the lemon garlic seasoning, onion, and butter.

Take the spaghetti squash and cook on high for hours.

Once cooked, remove the spaghetti squash from the Crockpot and run a fork through the meat to create the strands.

Take the squash strands back to the Crockpot and add the shrimps.

Season with pepper and salt.

Continue cooking on high for 30 minutes or until the shrimps have turned pink.

Nutrition:

Calories: 363.3

Carbohydrates: 1g

Protein: 33g

Fat: 21.2g

Cajun Seafood Pasta

Preparation Time: 15 minutes

Cooking Time: 16 minutes

Servings: 6

Ingredients:

- 2 cups thick whipped cream
- 1 tablespoon chopped fresh basil
- 1 tablespoon chopped fresh thyme
- 2 teaspoons salt
- 2 teaspoons ground black pepper
- 1 1/2 teaspoon ground red pepper flakes
- 1 teaspoon ground white pepper
- 1 cup chopped green onions
- 1 cup chopped parsley
- 1/2 shrimp, peeled
- 1/2 cup scallops
- 1/2 cup of grated Swiss cheese
- 1/2 cup grated Parmesan cheese
- 1 pound dry fettuccine pasta

Directions:

Cook the pasta in a large pot with boiling salted water until al dente.

Meanwhile, pour the cream into a large skillet. Cook over medium heat, constantly stirring until it boils. Reduce heat and add spices, salt, pepper, onions, and parsley. Let simmer for 7 to 8 minutes or until thick.

Stir seafood and cook until shrimp are no longer transparent. Stir in the cheese and mix well.

Drain the pasta. Serve the sauce over the noodles.

Nutrition:

695 calories

36.7 grams of fat

62.2 g carbohydrates

31.5 g of protein

193 mg cholesterol

1054of sodium

Tortellini in Red Pepper Sauce

Preparation time: 15 minutes

Cooking time: 10 minutes

Servings: 4

Ingredients:

- 1 (16-ounce) container fresh cheese tortellini (usually green and white pasta)
- 1 (16-ounce) jar roasted red peppers, drained
- 1 teaspoon garlic powder
- ¼ cup tahini
- 1 tablespoon red pepper oil (optional)

Directions:

1. Cook the tortellini according to package directions.
2. In a blender, combine the red peppers with the garlic powder and process until smooth.
3. Once blended, add the tahini until the sauce is thickened. If the sauce gets too thick, add up to 1 tablespoon red pepper oil (if using).
4. Once tortellini are cooked, drain and leave the pasta in a colander. Put the sauce to the bottom of the empty pot and heat for 2 minutes.
5. Then, add the tortellini back into the pot and cook for 2 more minutes. Serve and enjoy!

Nutrition:

Calories: 350

Protein: 12g

Carbohydrates: 46g

Sugars: 2g

Fiber: 4g

Fat: 11g

Linguine and Brussels Sprouts

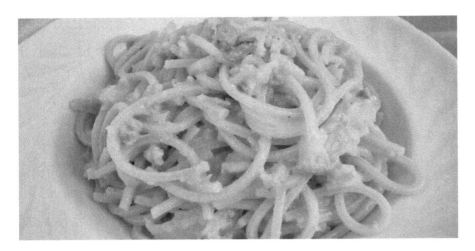

Preparation time: 15 minutes

Cooking time: 25 minutes

Servings: 4

Ingredients:

- 8 ounces whole-wheat linguine
- 1/3 cup + 2 tablespoons extra-virgin olive oil, divided
- 1 medium sweet onion, diced
- 2 to 3 garlic cloves, smashed
- 8 ounces Brussels sprouts, chopped
- 1/3 cup chicken stock, as needed
- 1/3 cup dry white wine
- ½ cup shredded Parmesan cheese
- 1 lemon, cut into quarters

Directions:

1. Cook the pasta according to package directions. Drain, and set aside 1 cup of the pasta water. Mix the cooked pasta with 2 tablespoons of olive oil, then set aside.

2. In a large sauté pan or skillet, heat the remaining 1/3 cup of olive oil on medium heat. Put the onion in the pan and cook for about 5 minutes, until softened. Put the smashed garlic cloves and cook for 1 minute, until fragrant.

3. Add the Brussels sprouts and cook covered for 15 minutes. Add chicken stock as needed to prevent burning. Once Brussels sprouts have wilted and are fork-tender, add white wine and cook down for about 7 minutes, until reduced.

4. Add the pasta to the skillet and add the pasta water as needed.

5. Serve with the Parmesan cheese and lemon for squeezing over the dish right before eating.

Nutrition:

Calories: 502

Protein: 15g

Carbohydrates: 50g

Sugars: 3g

Fiber: 9g

Fat: 31g

Creamy Chickpea Sauce with Whole-Wheat Fusilli

Preparation time: 15 minutes

Cooking time: 15 minutes

Servings: 4

Ingredients:

- ¼ cup extra-virgin olive oil
- ½ large shallot, chopped
- 5 garlic cloves, thinly sliced
- 1 (15-ounce) can chickpeas, drained and rinsed, reserving ½ cup canning liquid
- Pinch red pepper flakes
- 1 cup whole-grain fusilli pasta
- ¼ teaspoon salt
- 1/8 teaspoon freshly ground black pepper
- ¼ cup shaved fresh Parmesan cheese
- ¼ cup chopped fresh basil
- 2 teaspoons dried parsley
- 1 teaspoon dried oregano
- Red pepper flakes

Directions:

1. Warm-up the oil over medium heat in a medium pan and sauté the shallot and garlic for 3 to 5 minutes, until the garlic is golden. Add ¾ of the chickpeas plus 2 tablespoons of liquid from the can, and bring to a simmer.

2. Remove from the heat, transfer into a standard blender, and blend until smooth. At this point, add the remaining chickpeas. Add more reserved chickpea liquid if it becomes thick.

3. Boil the salted water in a pot and cook pasta until al dente, about 8 minutes. Reserve ½ cup of the pasta water, drain the pasta and return it to the pot.

4. Add the chickpea sauce to the hot pasta and add up to ¼ cup of the pasta water.

5. Put the pasta pot on medium heat and occasionally mix until the sauce thickens—season with salt and pepper.

6. Serve, garnished with parmesan, basil, parsley, oregano, and red pepper flakes.

Nutrition:

Calories: 310

Protein: 10g

Carbohydrates: 33g

Sugars: 1g

Fiber: 7g

Fat: 17g

Soups recipes

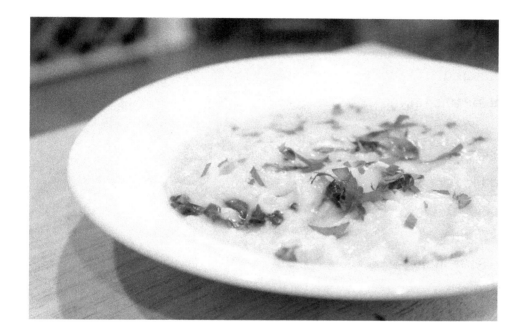

Roasted Pepper Soup

Preparation Time: 10 minutes

Cooking Time: 55 minutes

Servings: 4

Ingredients:

- 2 tomatoes, halved
- 3 red bell peppers, halved and deseeded
- 1 yellow onion, quartered
- 2 garlic cloves, peeled and halved
- 2 tablespoons olive oil
- 2 cups veggie stock
- A pinch of salt and black pepper
- 2 tablespoons tomato paste
- ¼ cup parsley, chopped
- ¼ teaspoon Italian seasoning
- ¼ teaspoon sweet paprika

Directions:

Spread the bell peppers, tomatoes, onion and garlic on a baking sheet lined with parchment paper, add oil, salt and pepper and bake at 375 degrees F for 45 minutes.

Heat up a pot with the stock over medium heat, add the roasted vegetables and the other ingredients, stir, bring to a simmer and cook for 10 minutes.

Blend the mix using an immersion blender, divide the soup into bowls and serve.

Nutrition:

Calories: 273

Protein: 5.6

Fat: 11.2

Carbs: 15.7

Italian Meatball Soup

Preparation Time: 10 minutes

Cooking Time: 45 minutes

Servings: 6

Ingredients:

- 1/2 cup parmesan cheese, grated (optional)
- 1 free-range egg
- 1 cup breadcrumbs, optional
- 2 tablespoons fresh parsley, minced
- 1 teaspoon dried oregano
- 1/2 teaspoon sea salt
- ½ teaspoon black pepper
- 3 tablespoons olive oil

For the soup:

- 2 quarts chicken broth or beef broth
- 3 tablespoons tomato paste
- 1 onion, diced
- 2 bay leaves
- 4-5 sprigs fresh thyme
- ½ teaspoon whole black peppercorns

To serve:

- Fresh parmesan cheese, grated
- 1-2 tablespoons fresh basil leaves, torn
- 1-2 tablespoons fresh parsley, chopped
- Salt and pepper, to taste

Directions:

1. Put all the meatball fixings except the oil into a medium bowl. Mix and form into meatballs.
2. Place the oil into a stockpot, place over medium heat and add the meatballs, browning on all sides.
3. Remove the meatballs from the pan. Add more oil to the pan if needed, and then add the onion. Cook for five minutes until soft.
4. Add the remaining soup ingredients, stir well then cook for 10 minutes.
5. Put the meatballs in the pan and simmer for a few minutes to warm through. Serve and enjoy.

Nutrition:

Calories: 331

Protein: 14.3g

Carbs: 14.4g

Fat: 30.3g

Tuscan White Bean Soup with Sausage and Kale

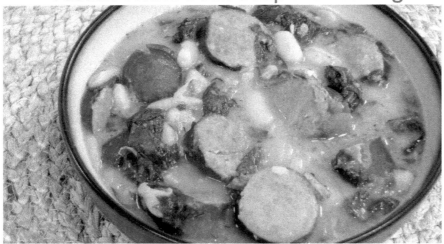

Preparation Time: 10 minutes

Cooking Time: 40 minutes

Servings: 6

Ingredients:

- ¼ cup extra virgin olive oil
- 1 lb. hot sausage,
- 1 onion, chopped
- 1 carrot, chopped
- 1 stalk celery, chopped
- 2 cloves garlic, chopped
- ½ lb. kale, stems removed and chopped
- 4 cups chicken broth
- 1 x 28 oz. can cannellini beans, rinsed and drained
- 1 teaspoon rosemary, dried

- 1 bay leaf

- ¼ teaspoon pepper

- Salt, to taste

- ½ cup shredded parmesan

Directions:

1. Find a stockpot, pop over medium heat, and add the oil.

2. Cook the sausage, then throw in the onion, carrot, celery, and garlic, then cook for a further five minutes. Add the kale and stir through.

3. Then add the broth, beans, rosemary, and bay leaf. Stir well, bring to the boil, then cover with the lid.

4. Turn down the heat, then simmer for 30 minutes. Serve and enjoy.

Nutrition:

Calories: 551

Protein: 36.3g

Carbs: 33.4g

Fat: 30.3g

Vegetable Soup

Preparation Time: 10 minutes

Cooking Time: 45 minutes

Servings: 4

Ingredients:

- Extra virgin olive oil, to taste
- 8 oz. sliced baby Bella mushrooms
- 2 medium-size zucchinis, sliced
- 1 bunch flat-leaf parsley, chopped
- 1 red onion, chopped
- 2 garlic cloves, chopped
- 2 celery ribs, chopped
- 2 carrots, peeled, chopped
- 2 golden potatoes, peeled, diced
- 1 teaspoon ground coriander
- 1/2 teaspoon turmeric powder
- 1/2 teaspoon sweet paprika
- 1/2 teaspoon thyme
- Salt and pepper
- 1 x 32 oz. can whole peeled tomatoes
- 2 bay leaves
- 6 cups turkey or vegetable broth
- 1 x 15 oz. can garbanzo beans, rinsed and drained

- Juice and zest of 1 lime

- 1/3 cup toasted pine nuts, optional

Directions:

1. Grab a large stockpot, add a tablespoon of olive oil, and pop over medium heat. Put the mushrooms and cook within five minutes, stirring often.

2. Remove, then put the sliced zucchini and cook for another five minutes. Remove from the pan.

3. Add more oil and add the parsley, onions, garlic, celery, carrots, and potatoes. Stir through the spices, salt, and pepper. Cook within five minutes until the veggies are softening.

4. Add the tomatoes, bay leaves, and broth, then boil. Cook on medium-low within 15 minutes.

5. Remove, then put the garbanzo beans, mushrooms and zucchini. Heat then serve and enjoy.

Nutrition:

Calories: 123

Protein: 12.3g

Carbs: 33.4g

Fat: 19.3g

Moroccan Lentil Soup

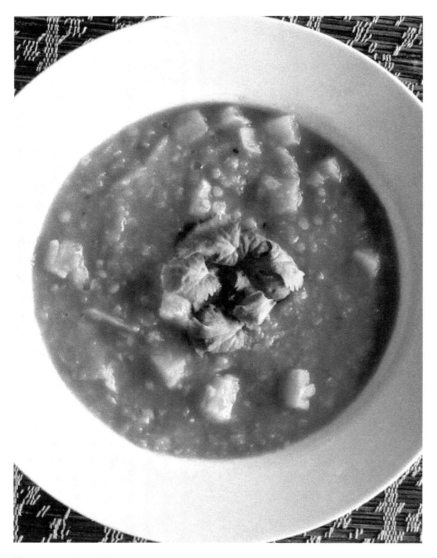

Preparation Time: 10 minutes

Cooking Time: 1 hour

Servings: 6

Ingredients:

- 2 tbsp extra virgin olive oil

- 1 large yellow onion, chopped

- 2 stalks celery, chopped

- 1 carrot, chopped

- 1/3 cup parsley, chopped

- 1/2 cup cilantro, chopped

- 5 large garlic cloves, minced
- 2"-piece ginger, minced
- 1 tsp ground turmeric
- 1 tsp ground cinnamon
- 2 tsp sweet paprika
- 1/2 tsp Aleppo pepper
- 1 & 1/4 cups dry red lentils
- 1 can garbanzo beans, drained
- 1 can sieve tomatoes
- 7–8 cups chicken broth or vegetable broth
- Coarse salt

To **Servings:**

- Dates
- Lemon wedges

Directions:

1. Grab a large saucepan, add the olive oil, and place over medium heat. Add the onion, celery, carrots, garlic, and ginger and cook for 5 minutes until soft.

2. Throw in the turmeric, cinnamon, paprika, and pepper and cook for another 5 minutes.

3. Add the tomatoes and broth, stir well then bring to a simmer. Add the lentils, garbanzo beans, cilantro, and parsley.

4. Cook uncovered for 35 minutes until the lentils become very soft. Season well, then serve and enjoy.

Nutrition:

Calories: 551

Protein: 36.3g

Carbs: 33.4g

Fat: 30.3g

Roasted Red Pepper and Tomato Soup

Preparation Time: 10 minutes

Cooking Time: 45 minutes

Servings: 4

Ingredients:

- 2 red bell peppers, seeded and halved
- 3 tomatoes, cored and halved
- 1/2 medium onion, quartered
- 2 cloves garlic, peeled and halved
- 1-2 tablespoons olive oil
- 1/4 teaspoon salt
- 1/4 teaspoon ground black pepper
- 2 cups vegetable broth
- 2 tablespoons tomato paste
- 1/4 cup fresh parsley, chopped
- 1/4 teaspoon Italian seasoning blend
- 1/4 teaspoon ground paprika
- 1/8 teaspoon. ground cayenne pepper, or more to taste

Directions:

1. Preheat your oven to 375°F.

2. Grab a medium bowl and add the red peppers, tomatoes, onion, garlic, olive oil, and salt and pepper. Toss well to coat.

3. Place onto a baking sheet and pop into the oven for 45 minutes until soft.

4. Then place the veggie broth over medium heat and add the roasted veggies, tomato paste, parsley, paprika, and cayenne. Mix, then simmer within 10 minutes.

5. Puree the soup in an immersion blender, then return to the pan. Reheat if required, add extra seasoning, then serve and enjoy.

Nutrition:

Calories: 531

Protein: 26.3g

Carbs: 33.4g

Fat: 30.3g

Greek Spring Soup

Preparation Time: 10 minutes

Cooking Time: 35 minutes

Servings: 4

Ingredients:

- 6 cups chicken broth
- 1 1/2 cups cooked chicken, shredded
- 2 tablespoons olive oil
- 1 small onion, diced
- 1 bay leaf
- 1/3 cup arborio rice
- 1 large free-range egg
- 2 tablespoons water
- Juice of half of a lemon
- 1 cup chopped asparagus
- 1 cup diced carrots
- 1/2 cup fresh chopped dill, divided
- Salt and pepper, to taste

Directions:

1. Find a large pan, add the oil, and place over medium heat. Add the onions and cook for five minutes until soft.

2. Then add ¼ cup dill, plus the chicken broth and bay leaf. Bring to a boil.

3. Add the rice and reduce the heat to low. Simmer for 10 minutes. Put the carrots and asparagus and cook for 10 more minutes until the rice and veggies are tender.

4. Add the chicken and simmer. Meanwhile, find a medium bowl and add the egg, lemon, and water. Whisk well.

5. Add ½ cup of the stock to the egg mixture, stirring constantly, then pour it all back into the pot.

6. Heat through and allow the soup to thicken. Add remaining dill, season well, then serve and enjoy.

Nutrition:

Calories: 551

Protein: 16.3g

Carbs: 23.4g

Fat: 10.3g

Minestrone Soup

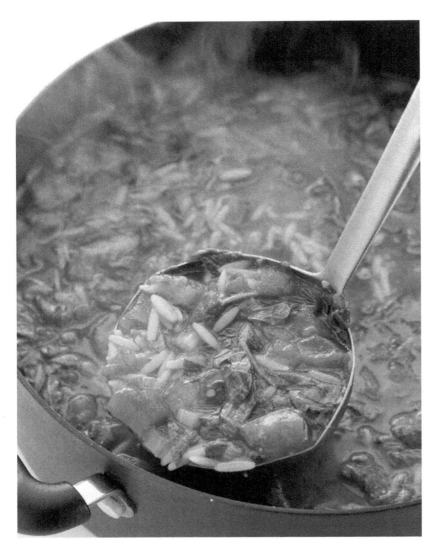

Preparation Time: 10 minutes

Cooking Time: 1 hour

Servings: 4

Ingredients:

- 1 small white onion, diced
- 4 cloves garlic, diced
- 1/2 cup carrots, sliced
- 1 medium zucchini, sliced
- 1 medium yellow squash, sliced

- 2 tablespoons minced fresh parsley
- 1/4 cup celery sliced
- 3 tablespoons olive oil
- 2 cans cannellini beans, drained
- 2 cans red kidney beans, drained
- 1 x 14.5 oz. can fire-roasted diced tomatoes, drained
- 4 cups vegetable stock
- 2 cups of water
- 1 1/2 teaspoons oregano
- 1/2 teaspoon basil
- 1/4 teaspoon thyme
- 1 teaspoon salt
- 1/2 teaspoon pepper
- 3/4 cup small pasta shells
- 4 cups fresh baby spinach
- 1/4 cup Parmesan or Romano cheese

Directions:

1. Grab a stockpot and place over medium heat. Add the oil, then the onions, garlic, carrots, zucchini, squash, parsley, and celery.

2. Cook for five minutes until the veggies are getting soft. Pour in the stock, water, beans, tomatoes, herbs, and salt and pepper. Stir well.

3. Reduce the heat, cover, and simmer for 30 minutes. Add the pasta and spinach, stir well, then cover and cook for a further 20 minutes until the pasta is cooked through.

4. Stir through the cheese, then serve and enjoy.

Nutrition:

Calories34

Protein: 26.3g

Carbs: 33.4g

Fat: 30.3g

Lemon Chicken Soup

Preparation Time: 10 minutes

Cooking Time: 20 minutes

Servings: 6

Ingredients:

- 10 cups chicken broth
- 3 tablespoons olive oil
- 8 cloves garlic, minced
- 1 sweet onion, sliced
- 1 large lemon, zested
- 2 boneless skinless chicken breasts
- 1 cup Israeli couscous
- 1/2 teaspoon crushed red pepper
- 2 oz. crumbled feta
- 1/3 cup chopped chive
- Salt and pepper, to taste

Directions:

1. Put the oil on medium heat in a pot, then put the onion and garlic and cook for five minutes until soft.

2. Add the broth, chicken breasts, lemon zest, and crushed pepper. Raise the heat, cover, and bring to a boil.

3. Reduce the heat, then simmer for 5 minutes. Remove, then pop onto a place and use two forks to shred. Pop back into the pot, add the feta, chives, and salt and pepper. Stir well, then serve and enjoy.

Nutrition:

Calories: 251

Protein: 16.3g

Carbs: 23.4g

Fat: 30.3g

Tuscan Vegetable Pasta Soup

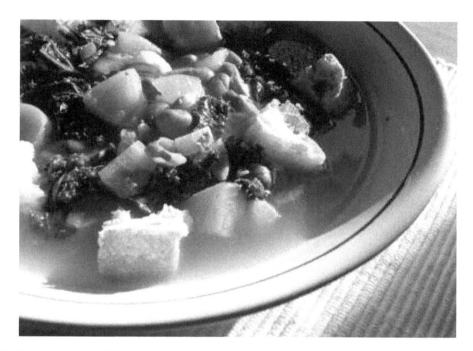

Preparation Time: 10 minutes

Cooking Time: 30 minutes

Servings: 6

Ingredients:

- 2 tablespoons extra virgin olive oil
- 4 cloves garlic, minced
- 1 medium yellow onion, diced
- 1/2 cup carrot, chopped
- 1/2 cup celery, chopped
- 1 medium zucchini, sliced and quartered
- 1 x 15 oz. can dice tomatoes
- 6 cups vegetable stock
- 2 tablespoons tomato paste
- 6-8 oz. whole wheat pasta
- 1 x 15 oz. can white beans
- 2 large handfuls of baby spinach
- 6 basil cubes
- Salt and pepper, to taste
- Fresh chopped parsley, for garnish

Directions:

1. Grab a stockpot, add the oil, and pop over medium heat. Put the onion plus the garlic and cook for five minutes until soft.

2. Throw in the carrots, celery, and zucchini and cook for an extra 5 minutes, stirring occasionally.

3. Add the tomato and salt and pepper and cook for 1-2 minutes. Add the veggies broth and tomato paste, stir well, then bring to the boil.

4. Throw in the pasta, cook for 10 minutes, then add the spinach, white beans, basil cubes, and seasoning.

5. Stir well, then remove from the heat. Divide between large bowls and serve and enjoy.

Nutrition:

Calories: 151

Protein: 26.3g

Carbs: 14.4g

Fat: 30.3g

Avgolemono Soup

Preparation Time: 10 minutes

Cooking time: 20 minutes

Servings: 6

Ingredients:

- 4 cups chicken stock
- 1 cup of water
- 1-pound chicken breast, shredded
- 1 cup of rice, cooked
- 3 egg yolks
- 3 tablespoons lemon juice
- 1/3 cup fresh parsley, chopped
- ½ teaspoon salt
- ¼ teaspoon ground black pepper

Directions:

1. Pour water and chicken stock into the saucepan and bring to boil. Then pour one cup of the hot liquid into the food processor.

2. Add cooked rice, egg yolks, lemon juice, and salt, then blend the mixture until smooth. After this, transfer the smooth rice mixture into the saucepan with the remaining chicken stock liquid.

3. Add shredded chicken breast, parsley, and ground black pepper. Boil the soup for 5 minutes more.

Nutrition:

Calories 235

Fat 5.6 g

Fiber 7.6g

Carbs 23.6 g

Protein 4.6 g

Italian Wedding Soup

Preparation time: 15 minutes

Cooking time: 40 minutes

Servings: 6

Ingredients:

- 1 lb. lean ground beef
- 1/3 cup breadcrumbs
- 1 egg, lightly beaten
- 1 onion, grated
- 2 carrots, chopped
- 1 small head escarole, 1/2-inch strips
- 1 cup baby spinach leaves
- 1/2 cup small pasta
- 2 tbsp Parmesan cheese, grated
- 2 tbsp parsley, finely cut
- 1 tsp salt
- 1 tsp ground black pepper
- 3 tbsp olive oil
- 3 cups chicken broth
- 3 cups of water
- 1 tsp oregano

Directions:

1. Combine ground beef, egg, onion, breadcrumbs, cheese, parsley, 1/2 teaspoon of salt, and 1/2 teaspoon of black pepper. Mix well with hands.

2. Using a tablespoon, make walnut-sized meatballs—warm olive oil in a large skillet and brown meatballs in batches. Place aside on a plate.

3. Boil broth and water, with carrots, oregano, and the remaining salt and pepper in a large soup pot. Gently add the meatballs.

4. Reduce heat and simmer for 30 minutes. Add pasta, spinach, and escarole and simmer for 10 more minutes.

Nutrition:

Calories: 370

Carbs: 26g

Fat: 21g

Protein: 20g

Lentil and Beef Soup

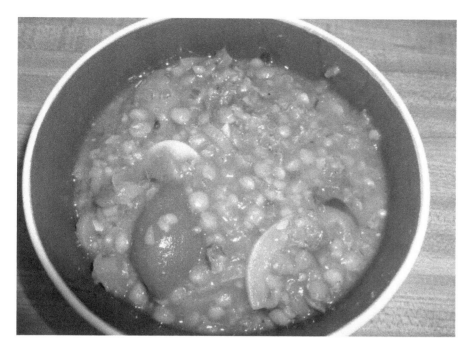

Preparation time: 15 minutes

Cooking time: 60 minutes

Servings: 6

Ingredients:

- 1 lb. ground beef
- 1 cup brown lentils
- 2 carrots, chopped
- 2 onions, chopped
- 1 potato, cut into 1/2-inch cubes
- 4 garlic cloves, chopped
- 2 tomatoes, grated or pureed

- 5 cups of water

- 1 tsp savory

- 1 tsp oregano

- 1 tsp paprika

- 2 tbsp olive oil

- 1 tsp salt

- black pepper, to taste

Directions:

1. Warm-up olive oil in a large soup pot. Brown beef, breaking it up with a spoon. Add paprika and garlic and stir. Add lentils, the remaining vegetables, water, and spice.

2. Bring to the boil. Reduce heat to low and simmer, covered, for about an hour, or until lentils are tender. Stir occasionally.

Nutrition:

Calories: 69

Carbs: 8g

Fat: 2g

Protein: 4g

Beef and Vegetable Soup

Preparation time: 15 minutes

Cooking time: 20 minutes

Servings: 8

Ingredients:

- 2 lbs. stewing beef
- 3 tbsp olive oil
- 1 large onion, chopped
- 4-5 white button mushrooms, chopped
- 2 carrots, chopped
- 1 celery rib, chopped
- 1/2 cup dry white wine
- 6 cups of water
- 2 tbsp tomato paste
- 1/2 cup parsley, chopped
- salt and black pepper, to taste

Directions:

1. Rub the beef pieces with salt plus pepper. Warm olive oil and seal the beef in batches in a large soup pot, then set it aside, covered.

2. Cook the onions, mushrooms, carrots, and celery over medium-high heat. Add the wine, stir, and return the meat to the pot.

3. Add water and bring to a boil. Simmer, covered, within an hour, mixing occasionally.

4. Put the tomato paste in a few tablespoons of the soup and add it to the pot. Stir in the chopped parsley and season with salt and pepper to taste.

Nutrition:

Calories: 120

Carbs: 17g

Fat: 3g

Protein: 7g

Beef and Vegetable Minestrone

Preparation time: 15 minutes

Cooking time: 35 minutes

Servings: 7

Ingredients:

- 2 slices bacon, chopped
- 1 cup ground beef
- 2 carrots, chopped
- 2 cloves garlic, finely chopped
- 1 large onion, chopped
- 1 celery rib, chopped
- 1 can tomatoes, chopped
- 6 cups beef broth
- 1 can chickpeas, drained
- 1/2 cup small pasta
- 1 bay leaf
- 1 tsp dried basil
- 1 tsp dried rosemary
- 1/4 tsp crushed chilies

Directions:

1. Cook bacon plus ground beef in a large saucepan, breaking up the beef as it cooks. Drain off the fat and add carrots, garlic, onion, and celery.

2. Cook for about five minutes or until the onions are translucent. Season with basil, bay leaf, rosemary, and crushed chilies. Stir in the tomatoes and beef broth.

3. Boil then simmer within 20 minutes. Add in the chickpeas and pasta. Cook, uncovered, within 10 minutes, or until the pasta is ready.

Nutrition:

Calories: 100

Carbs: 20g

Fat: 2g

Protein: 4g

Bean, Chicken and Sausage Soup

Preparation time: 15 minutes

Cooking time: 40 minutes

Servings: 8

Ingredients:

- 10.5 oz Italian sausage
- 3 bacon strips, diced
- 2 cups chicken, cooked and diced
- 1 cup canned beans, rinsed and drained
- 1 big onion, chopped
- 2 garlic cloves, pressed
- 3 cups of water
- 1 cup canned tomatoes, diced, undrained
- 1 bay leaf
- 1 tsp dried thyme
- 1 tsp savory
- 1/2 tsp dried basil
- salt and pepper, to taste

Directions:

1. Cook the sausage, onion, and bacon over medium heat until the sausage is no longer pink. Drain off the fat.

2. Add the garlic and cook for a minute. Add the water, tomatoes, and seasonings and bring to a boil.

3. Cover, reduce heat and simmer for 30 minutes. Add chicken and beans. Simmer for 5 minutes more and serve.

Nutrition:

Calories: 196

Carbs: 7g

Fat: 12g

Protein: 15g

Moroccan Chicken and Butternut Squash Soup

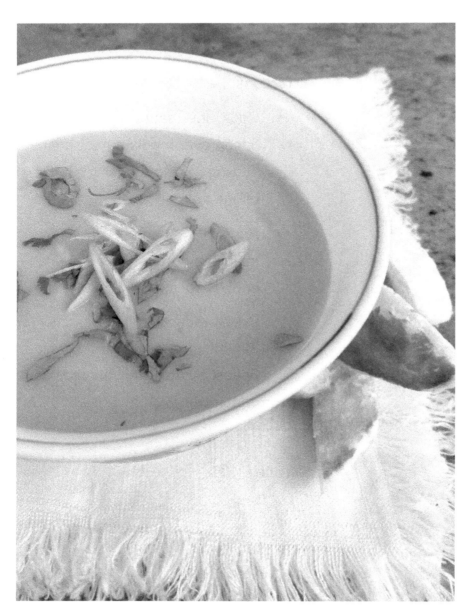

Preparation time: 15 minutes

Cooking time: 20 minutes

Servings: 8

Ingredients:

- 3 skinless, boneless chicken thighs, bite-sized
- 1 big onion, chopped
- 1 zucchini, sliced into 1/2-inch pieces
- 3 cups butternut squash
- 2 tbsp tomato paste
- 4 cups chicken broth
- 1/3 cup uncooked couscous
- 1/2 tsp ground cumin
- 1/4 tsp ground cinnamon
- 1 tsp paprika
- 1 tsp salt
- 2 tbsp fresh basil, chopped
- 1 tbsp grated orange rind
- 3 tbsp olive oil

Directions:

1. Heat a soup pot over medium heat. Gently sauté onion for 3-4 minutes, stirring occasionally.

2. Add chicken pieces and cook for 5 minutes until chicken is brown on all sides. Add cumin, cinnamon, and paprika and stir well.

3. Add butternut squash and tomato paste; stir again. Add chicken broth and bring to a boil, then reduce heat and simmer for 10 minutes.

4. Stir in couscous, salt, and zucchini pieces; cook until squash is tender. Remove pot from heat—season with salt and pepper to taste. Stir in chopped basil and orange rind and serve.

Nutrition:

Calories: 292

Carbs: 31g

Fat: 8g

Protein: 24g

Chicken Soup with Vermicelli

Preparation time: 15 minutes

Cooking time: 30 minutes

Servings: 4

Ingredients:

- 1 whole chicken leg or 1/2 lb. chicken breast
- 1/2 cup vermicelli
- 1 carrot, grated
- 4 cups of water
- 3 cloves of garlic, sliced
- 1 tsp salt
- 1/2 tsp black pepper
- 1 egg, beaten
- 2 tbsp lemon juice

Directions:

1. Arrange the chicken in a pot, then add 4 cups of water. Add 1 teaspoon salt and boil until the chicken is cooked. Take the chicken out of the pot, let it cool a little, and cut it into bite-size pieces.

2. Add carrot and garlic to the soup and bring it to a boil. Add vermicelli and chicken pieces. Simmer over medium heat for 8-10 minutes.

3. Mix the beaten egg plus lemon juice in a bowl and slowly stir into the soup. Do not boil it again. Serve soup warm, seasoned with black pepper to taste.

Nutrition:

Calories: 400

Carbs: 48g

Fat: 15g

Protein: 18g

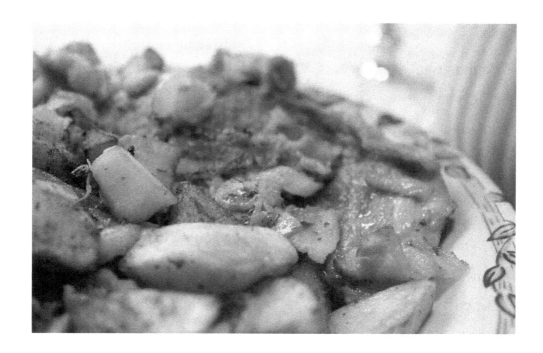

Crockpot Beef Stroganoff

Preparation Time: 30 minutes

Cooking Time: 8 hours

Servings: 8

Ingredients:

- 2-pounds beef stew meat
- 2 tsps. salt
- ½ tsp. black pepper
- 1 tsp. garlic powder
- 3 tbsps. EVOO
- 2 tsps. paprika
- 1 tsp. thyme
- 1 tsp. onion powder
- 8 ounces mushrooms, sliced
- 1 small onion, sliced
- 1/3 c. coconut cream
- 2 tsps. vinegar

Directions:

Season the beef stew meat with pepper and salt. Add the garlic powder, oil, paprika, thyme, and onion powder. Stir to mix all ingredients. Let the beef marinate for 2 hours inside the fridge.

Take the mushrooms and onion in the Crockpot and Take the seasoned beef on top.

Close the lid and then cook on low for 8 hours.

Once the meat is nearly done, add the coconut cream and vinegar. Adjust the seasoning if needed.

Nutrition:

Calories: 381

Carbohydrates: 2g

Protein: 27.9g

Fat: 24.5g

Pork Stew with Oyster Mushrooms

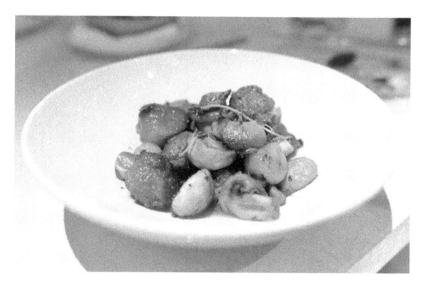

Preparation Time: 25 minutes

Cooking Time: 1o hours

Servings: 4

Ingredients:

- 2 tbsp. coconut oil
- medium onion, chopped
- 1 clove of garlic, chopped
- 2 pounds pork loin, cut into cubes
- Pepper and salt to taste
- 2 tbsps. oregano
- 2 tbsps. dried mustard
- ½ tsp. ground nutmeg
- 1 ½ c. bone broth
- 2 pounds oyster mushroom, rinsed
- ¼ c. full fat coconut milk
- ¼ c. ghee
- 3 tbsp. capers

Directions:

Cook the coconut oil in a pan on medium flame. Sauté the onion and garlic until fragrant. Add the pork loin and brown all sides. Season with pepper and salt to taste.

Transfer the sautéed meat, garlic, and onions in the Crockpot.

Add the oregano, mustard, nutmeg, bone broth, and oyster mushrooms.

Give a stir and cook on low for 10 hours.

Before the meat is nearly cooked, add the coconut milk and ghee.

Once done cooking, garnish with capers.

Nutrition:

Calories: 734

Carbohydrates: 12.5g

Protein: 50.4g

Fat: 48.9g

Easy Crockpot Pork Loin

Preparation Time: 40 minutes

Cooking Time: 10 hours

Servings: 12

Ingredients:

- 5 pounds pork loin
- Pepper and salt to taste
- 2 onions, chopped
- 3 c. beef broth

Directions:

Season the pork loin with pepper and salt.

Take inside the Crockpot and arrange the onions around the roast.

Pour the beef broth.

Cook on low for 10 hours until tender.

Nutrition:

Calories: 372

Carbohydrates: 0g

Protein: 37.5g

Fat: 23.4g

Braised Short Ribs with Red Wine

Preparation Time: 10 minutes

Cooking Time: 1-2 hours

Servings: 4

Ingredients:

- 1½ pounds boneless beef short ribs (if using bone-in, use 3½ pounds)
- 1 teaspoon salt
- ½ teaspoon freshly ground black pepper
- ½ teaspoon garlic powder
- ¼ cup extra-virgin olive oil
- 1 cup of dry red wine (abernet sauvignon or merlot)
- 2 to 3 cups beef broth, divided
- 4 sprigs rosemary

Directions:

Preheat the oven to 350°F.

Rub the short ribs with pepper, salt, and garlic powder. Let sit for 10 minutes.

In a Dutch oven or oven-safe deep skillet, heat the olive oil on medium-high heat.

When the oil becomes very hot, add now the short ribs and brown until dark in color, 2 to 3 minutes per side. Remove the meat from the oil and keep warm.

Add the red wine and 2 cups beef broth to the Dutch oven, whisk together, and bring to boil. Lessen the heat and let it simmer until the liquid is reduced to about 2 cups, about 10 minutes.

Return the short ribs to the liquid, which should come about halfway up the meat, adding up to 1 cup of remaining broth if needed. Cover and braise until the meat is very tender, about 1½ to 2 hours.

Remove it from the oven and then let sit, covered, for 10 minutes before serving. Serve warm, drizzled with cooking liquid.

Nutrition:

Calories: 792

Carbohydrates: 2g

Protein: 25g

Fat: 76g

Lamb Kofte with Yogurt Sauce

Preparation Time: 30 minutes + 10 minutes to rest

Cooking Time: 15 minutes

Servings: 4

Ingredients:

- 1-pound ground lamb
- ½ cup chopped fresh mint + 2 tablespoons
- ¼ cup almond or coconut flour
- ¼ cup finely chopped red onion
- ¼ cup toasted pine nuts
- 2 teaspoons ground cumin
- 1½ teaspoons salt, divided
- 1 teaspoon ground cinnamon
- 1 teaspoon ground ginger
- ½ teaspoon ground nutmeg
- ½ teaspoon freshly ground black pepper
- 1 cup plain whole-milk Greek yogurt
- 2 tablespoons extra-virgin olive oil
- Zest and juice of 1 lime

Directions:

Heat the oven broiler to the low setting. You can also bake these at high heat (450 to 475°F) if you happen to have a very hot broiler. Submerge four wooden skewers in water and let soak at least 10 minutes to prevent them from burning.

In a large bowl, combine the lamb, ½ cup mint, almond flour, red onion, pine nuts, cumin, 1 teaspoon salt, cinnamon, ginger, nutmeg, and pepper and, using your hands, incorporate all the ingredients together well.

Form the mixture into 12 egg-shaped patties and let sit for 10 minutes.

Remove the skewers from the water, thread 3 patties onto each skewer, and place on a pan or wire rack on top of a baking sheet lined with aluminum foil. Broil on the top rack until golden and cooked through, 8 to 12 minutes, flipping once halfway through cooking.

Combine the yogurt, olive oil, remaining 2 tablespoons chopped mint, remaining ½ teaspoon salt, and lime zest and juice and whisk to combine well. Keep cool until ready to use.

Serve the skewers with yogurt sauce.

Nutrition:

Calories: 500

Carbohydrates: 9g

Protein: 23g

Fat: 42g

Mediterranean Pork Roast

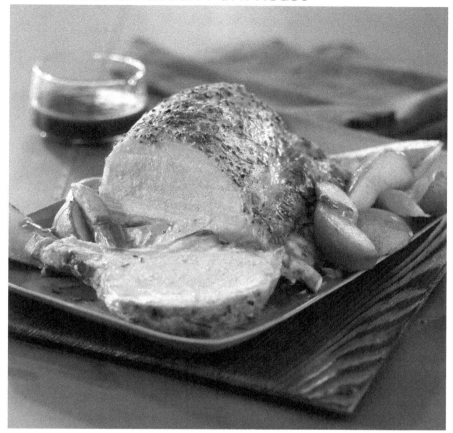

Preparation Time: 10 minutes

Cooking Time: 8 hours and 10 minutes

Servings: 6

Ingredients:

- Olive oil - 2 tablespoons
- Pork roast - 2 pounds
- Paprika - ½ teaspoon
- Chicken broth - ¾ cup
- Dried sage - 2 teaspoons
- Garlic minced - ½ tablespoon
- Dried marjoram - ¼ teaspoon
- Dried Rosemary - ¼ teaspoon
- Oregano - 1 teaspoon
- Dried thyme - ¼ teaspoon
- Basil - 1 teaspoon
- Kosher salt - ½ teaspoon

Directions:

In a small bowl mix broth, oil, salt, and spices.

In a skillet pour olive oil and bring to medium-high heat.

Put the pork into it and roast until all sides become brown.

Take out the pork after cooking and poke the roast all over with a knife.

Place the poked pork roast into a 6-quart crock pot.

Now, pour the small bowl mixture liquid all over the roast.

Close the crock pot and cook on low heat setting for 8 hours.

After cooking, remove it from the crock pot on to a cutting board and shred into pieces.

Afterward, add the shredded pork back into the crockpot.

Simmer it another 10 minutes.

Serve along with feta cheese, pita bread, and tomatoes.

Nutrition:

Calories: 361

Carbohydrate: 0.7g

Protein: 43.8g

Sugars: 0.1g

Fat: 10.4g

Dietary Fiber: 0.3g

Cholesterol: 130mg

Sodium: 374mg

Potassium: 647mg

Beef, Artichoke & Mushroom Stew

Preparation Time: 20 minutes

Cooking Time: 2 hours and 15 minutes

Servings: 6

Ingredients:

For Beef Marinade:

- 1 onion, chopped
- 1 garlic clove, crushed
- 2 tablespoons fresh thyme, hopped
- ½ cup dry red wine
- 2 tablespoons tomato puree
- 2 tablespoons olive oil
- 1 teaspoon cayenne pepper
- Pinch of salt and ground black pepper
- 1½ pounds beef stew meat, cut into large chunks

For Stew:

- 2 tablespoons olive oil
- 2 tablespoons all-purpose flour
- ½ cup water
- ½ cup dry red wine

- 12 ounces jar artichoke hearts, drained and cut into small chunks
- 4 ounces button mushrooms, sliced
- Salt and ground black pepper, as required

Directions:

For marinade: in a large bowl, add all the ingredients except the beef and mix well.

Add the beef and coat with the marinade generously.

Refrigerate to marinate overnight.

Remove the beef from bowl, reserving the marinade.

In a large pan, heat the oil and sear the beef in 2 batches for about 5 minutes or until browned.

With a slotted spoon, transfer the beef into a bowl.

In the same pan, add the reserved marinade, flour, water and wine and stir to combine.

Stir in the cooked beef and bring to a boil.

Reduce the heat to low and simmer, covered for about 2 hours, stirring occasionally.

Stir in the artichoke hearts and mushrooms and simmer for about 30 minutes.

Stir in the salt and black pepper and bring to a boil over high heat.

Remove from the eat ad serve hot.

Nutrition:

Calories 367

Total Fat 16.6 g

Saturated Fat 4 g

Cholesterol 101 mg

Total Carbs 9.6 g

Sugar 2.2 g

Fiber 3.1 g

Sodium 292 mg

Potassium 624 mg

Protein 36.7 g

Beef & Tapioca Stew

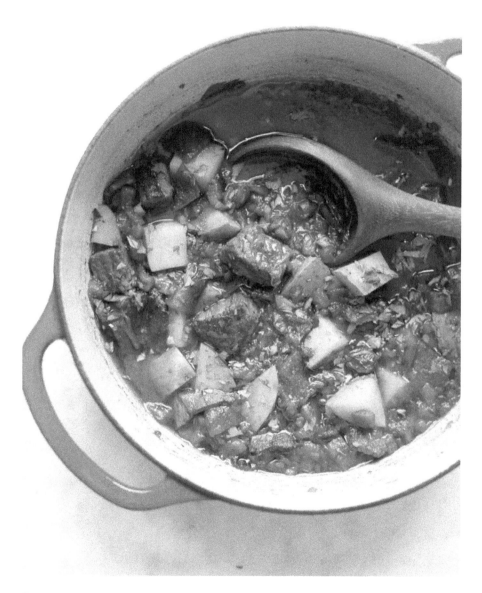

Preparation Time: *20 minutes*

Cooking Time: *1 hour and 45 minutes*

Servings: 8

Ingredients:

- 1 tablespoon olive oil
- 2 pounds boneless beef chuck roast, cut into ¾-inch cubes
- 1 (14½-ounce) can diced tomatoes with juice
- ¼ cup quick-cooking tapioca
- 1 tablespoon honey
- 2 teaspoons ground cinnamon
- ¼ teaspoon garlic powder
- Ground black pepper, as required
- ¼ cup red wine vinegar
- 2 cups beef broth
- 3 cups sweet potato, peeled and cubed
- 2 medium onions, cut into thin wedges
- 2 cups prunes, pitted

Directions:

In a Dutch oven, heat 1 tablespoon of oil over medium-high heat and sear the beef cubes in 2 batches for bout 4-5 minutes or until browned.

Drain off the grease from the pan.

Stir in the tomatoes, tapioca, honey, cinnamon, garlic powder, black pepper, vinegar and broth and bring to a boil.

Reduce the heat to low and simmer, covered for about 1 hour, stirring occasionally.

Stir in the onions and sweet potato and simmer, covered for about 20-30 minutes.

Stir in the prunes and cook for about 3-5 minutes.

Serve hot.

Nutrition:

Calories 675

Total Fat34. 1 g

Saturated Fat 13 g

Cholesterol 117 mg

Total Carbs 59.6 g

Sugar 26 g

Fiber 7.1 g

Sodium 295 mg

Potassium 1150 mg

Protein 34.1 g

Beef Pizza

Preparation Time: *20 minutes*

Cooking Time: *50 minutes*

Servings: 10

Ingredients:

- For Crust:
- 3 cups all-purpose flour
- 1 tablespoon sugar
- 2¼ teaspoons active dry yeast
- 1 teaspoon salt
- 2 tablespoons olive oil
- 1 cup warm water
- For Topping:
- 1-pound ground beef
- 1 medium onion, chopped
- 2 tablespoons tomato paste
- 1 tablespoon ground cumin
- Salt and ground black pepper, as required
- ¼ cup water
- 1 cup fresh spinach, chopped
- 8 ounces artichoke hearts, quartered
- 4 ounces fresh mushrooms, sliced
- 2 tomatoes, chopped
- 4 ounces feta cheese, crumbled

Directions:

For crust: in the bowl of a stand mixer, fitted with the dough hook, add the flour, sugar, yeast and salt.

Add 2 tablespoons of the oil and warm water and knead until a smooth and elastic dough is formed.

Make a ball of the dough and set aside for about 15 minutes.

Place the dough onto a lightly floured surface and roll into a circle.

Place the dough into a lightly, greased round pizza pan and gently, press to fit.

Set aside for about 10-15 minutes.

Coat the crust with some oil.

Preheat the oven to 400 degrees F.

For topping: heat a nonstick skillet over medium-high heat and cook the beef for about 4-5 minutes.

Add the onion and cook for about 5 minutes, stirring frequently.

Add the tomato paste, cumin, salt, black pepper and water and stir to combine.

125

Reduce the heat to medium and cook for about 5-10 minutes.

Remove from the heat and set aside.

Place the beef mixture over the pizza crust and top with the spinach, followed by the artichokes, mushrooms, tomatoes, and Feta cheese.

Bake for about 25-30 minutes or until the cheese is melted.

Remove from the oven and set aside for about 3-5 minutes before slicing.

Cut into desired sized slices and serve.

Nutrition:

Calories 309

Total Fat 8.7 g

Saturated Fat 3.3 g

Cholesterol 51 mg

Total Carbs 36.4 g

Sugar 3.7 g

Fiber 3.3 g

Sodium 421 mg

Potassium 502 mg

Protein 21.4 g

Beef & Bulgur Meatballs

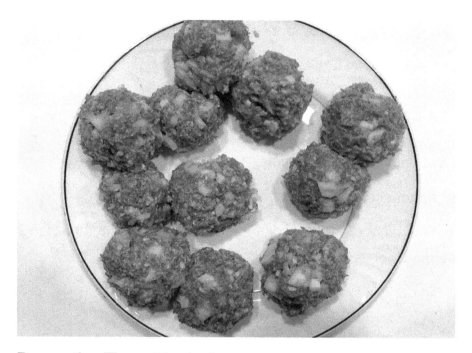

Preparation Time: *20 minutes*

Cooking Time: *28 minutes*

Servings: 6

Ingredients:

- ¾ cup uncooked bulgur
- 1-pound ground beef
- ¼ cup shallots, minced
- ¼ cup fresh parsley, minced
- ½ teaspoon ground allspice
- ½ teaspoon ground cumin
- ½ teaspoon ground cinnamon
- ¼ teaspoon red pepper flakes, crushed
- Salt, as required

- 1 tablespoon olive oil

Directions:

In a large bowl of the cold water, soak the bulgur for about 30 minutes.

Drain the bulgur well and then, squeeze with your hands to remove the excess water.

In a food processor, add the bulgur, beef, shallot, parsley, spices and salt and pulse until a smooth mixture is formed.

Transfer the mixture into a bowl and refrigerate, covered for about 30 minutes.

Remove from the refrigerator and make equal sized balls from the beef mixture.

In a large nonstick skillet, heat the oil over medium-high heat and cook the meatballs in 2 batches for about 13-14 minutes, flipping frequently.

Serve warm.

Nutrition:

Calories 228

Total Fat 7.4 g

Saturated Fat 2.2 g

Cholesterol 68 mg

Total Carbs 15 g

Sugar 0.1 g

Fiber 3.5 g

Sodium 83 mg

Potassium 420 mg

Protein 25.4 g

Tasty Beef and Broccoli

Preparation Time: *10 minutes*

Cooking Time: *15 minutes*

Servings: *4*

Ingredients:

- 1 and ½ pounds flanks steak, cut into thin strips
- 1 tablespoon olive oil
- 1 tablespoon tamari sauce
- 1 cup beef stock
- 1 pound broccoli, florets separated

Directions:

In a bowl, mix steak strips with oil and tamari, toss and leave aside for 10 minutes.

Set your instant pot on sauté mode, add beef strips and brown them for 4 minutes on each side.

Add stock, stir, cover pot again and cook on high for 8 minutes.

Add broccoli, stir, cover pot again and cook on high for 4 minutes more.

Divide everything between plates and serve.

Enjoy!

Nutrition:

Calories: 312

Protein: 4 g

Fat: 5 g

Carbohydrates: 20 g

Beef Corn Chili

Preparation Time: *8-10 minutes*

Cooking Time: *30 minutes*

Servings: 8

Ingredients:

- 2 small onions, chopped (finely)
- ¼ cup canned corn
- 1 tablespoon oil
- 10 ounces lean ground beef
- 2 small chili peppers, diced

Directions:

Take your instant pot and place over dry kitchen surface; open its top lid and switch it on.

Press. "SAUTE".

In its Cooking pot, add and heat the oil.

Add the onions, chili pepper, and beef; cook for 2-3 minutes until turn translucent and softened.

Add the 3 cups water in the Cooking pot; combine to mix well.

Close its top lid and make sure that its valve it closed to avoid spilling.

Press "MEAT/STEW". Adjust the timer to 20 minutes.

Press will slowly build up; let the added ingredients to cook until the timer indicates zero.

Press "CANCEL". Now press "NPR" for natural release pressure. Instant pot will gradually release pressure for about 8-10 minutes.

Open the top lid; transfer the cooked recipe in serving plates.

Serve the recipe warm.

Nutrition:

Calories: 94

Protein: 7 g

Fat: 5 g

Carbohydrates: 2 g

Balsamic Beef Dish

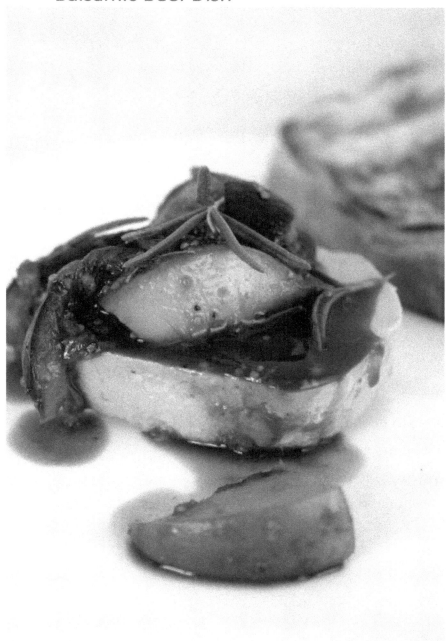

Preparation Time: *5 minutes*

Cooking Time: *55 minutes*

Servings: 8

Ingredients:

- 3 pounds chuck roast
- 3 cloves garlic, thinly sliced
- 1 tablespoon oil
- 1 teaspoon flavored vinegar
- ½ teaspoon pepper
- ½ teaspoon rosemary
- 1 tablespoon butter
- ½ teaspoon thyme
- ¼ cup balsamic vinegar
- 1 cup beef broth

Directions:

Cut slits in the roast and stuff garlic slices all over.

Take a bowl and add flavored vinegar, rosemary, pepper, thyme and rub the mixture over the roast.

Set your pot to sauté mode and add oil, allow the oil to heat up.

Add roast and brown both sides (5 minutes each side).

Take the roast out and keep it on the side.

Add butter, broth, balsamic vinegar and deglaze the pot.

Transfer the roast back and lock up the lid, cook on HIGH pressure for 40 minutes.

Perform a quick release.

Remove the lid and serve!

Nutrition:

Calories: 393

Protein: 37 g

Fat: 15 g

Carbohydrates: 25 g

Soy Sauce Beef Roast

Preparation Time: *8 minutes*

Cooking Time: 3*5 minutes*

Servings: 2-3

Ingredients:

- ½ teaspoon beef bouillon
- 1 ½ teaspoon rosemary
- ½ teaspoon minced garlic
- 2 pounds roast beef
- 1/3 cup soy sauce

Directions:

Mix the soy sauce, bouillon, rosemary, and garlic together in a mixing bowl.

Place your instant pot over as dry kitchen platform. Open the top lid and plug it on.

Add the roast, bowl mix and enough water to cover the roast; gently stir to mix well.

Properly close the top lid; make sure that the safety valve is properly locked.

Press "MEAT/STEW" Cooking function; set pressure level to "HIGH" and set the Cooking time to 35 minutes.

Allow the pressure to build to cook the ingredients.

After Cooking time is over press "CANCEL" setting. Find and press "NPR" Cooking function. This setting is for the natural release of inside pressure, and it takes around 10 minutes to release pressure slowly.

Slowly open the lid, take out the cooked meat and shred it.

Add the shredded meat back in the potting mix and stir to mix well.

Take out the cooked recipe in serving containers. Serve warm.

Nutrition:

Calories: 423

Protein: 21g

Fat: 14g

Carbohydrates: 12g

Rosemary Beef Chuck Roast

Preparation Time: *5 minutes*

Cooking Time: *45 minutes*

Servings: *5-6*

Ingredients:

- 3 pounds chuck beef roast
- 3 garlic cloves
- ¼ cup balsamic vinegar
- 1 sprig fresh rosemary
- 1 sprig fresh thyme
- 1 cup of water
- 1 tablespoon vegetable oil
- Salt and pepper to taste

Directions:

Cut slices in the beef roast and place the garlic cloves in them.

Coat the roast with the herbs, black pepper, and salt.

Preheat your instant pot using the sauté setting and add the oil.

When warmed, add the beef roast and stir-cook until browned on all sides.

Add the remaining ingredients; stir gently.

Seal the lid and cook on high pressure for 40 minutes using the manual setting.

Let the pressure release naturally, about 10 minutes.

Uncover the instant pot; transfer the beef roast the serving plates, slice and serve.

Nutrition:

Calories: 542

Protein: 55.2 g

Fat: 11.2 g

Carbohydrates: 8.7 g

Pork Chops and Tomato Sauce:

Preparation Time: *10 minutes*

Cooking Time: *20 minutes*

Servings: *4*

Ingredients:

- 4 pork chops, boneless
- 1 tablespoon soy sauce
- ¼ teaspoon sesame oil
- 1 and ½ cups tomato paste
- 1 yellow onion
- 8 mushrooms, sliced

Directions:

In a bowl, mix pork chops with soy sauce and sesame oil, toss and leave aside for 10 minutes.

Set your instant pot on sauté mode, add pork chops and brown them for 5 minutes on each side.

Add onion, stir and cook for 1-2 minutes more.

Add tomato paste and mushrooms, toss, cover and cook on high for 8-9 minutes.

Divide everything between plates and serve.

Enjoy!

Nutrition:

Calories: 300

Protein: 4 g

Fat: 7 g

Carbohydrates: 18 g

Pork Potato

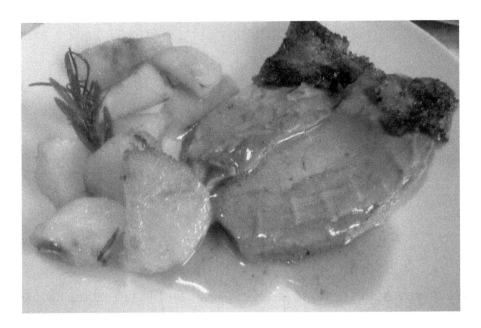

Preparation Time: *8-10 minutes*

Cooking Time: *25 minutes*

Servings: *4*

Ingredients:

- 10 ounces pork neck, fat remove and make small pieces
- 1 medium sweet potato, chopped
- 1 tablespoon oil
- 3 cups beef stock, Low – sodium
- 1 onion, chopped (finely)

Directions:

Take your pot and place over dry kitchen surface; open its top lid and switch it on.

Press "sauté". Grease the pot with some Cooking oil.

Add the onions; cook for 2 minutes until turn translucent and softened.

Add the meat; stir-cook for 4-5 minutes to evenly brown.

Mix in the stock and potatoes.

Close its top lid and make sure that its valve it closed to avoid spillage.

Press "Manual". Adjust the timer to 20 minutes.

Pressure will slowly build up; let the added ingredients to cook until the timer indicates zero.

Press "CANCEL". Now press "NPR" for natural release pressure. Instant pot will gradually release pressure for about 8-10 minutes.

Open the top lid transfer the cooked recipe in serving plates.

Serve the recipe warm.

Nutrition:

Calories: 278

Protein: 18 g

Fat: 18 g

Carbohydrates: 12 g

Coffee Flavored Pork Ribs

Preparation Time: *3 minutes*

Cooking Time: 40 *minutes*

Servings: *4*

Ingredients:

- 1 rack baby back ribs
- 2 teaspoons sesame oil
- 3 tablespoons oyster sauce
- 1 teaspoon salt
- 1 teaspoon sugar
- 1 cup of water
- A ½ cup of liquid smoke
- 2 tablespoons instant coffee powder

Directions:

Add the listed ingredients to the pot.

Lock the lid and cook on MEAT/STEW mode for 40 minutes.

Release the pressure naturally over 10 minutes.

Serve and enjoy!

Nutrition:

Calories: 898

Protein: 77 g

Fat: 63 g

Carbohydrates: 4 g

Tomato Pork Paste

Preparation Time: 5-8 *minutes*

Cooking Time: *15 minutes*

Servings: 4

Ingredients:

- 2 cups tomato puree
- 1 tablespoon red wine
- 1 pound lean ground pork
- 8-10 ounce pack paste of your choice, uncooked
- Salt and black pepper to taste
- 1 tablespoon vegetable oil

Directions:

Season the pork with black pepper and salt.

Place your instant pot over a dry kitchen platform. Open the top lid and plug it on.

Press "SAUTE" Cooking function; add the oil and heat it.

In the pot, add the ground meat; stir-cook using wooden spatula until turns evenly brown for 8-10 minutes.

Add the wine. Cook for 1-2 minutes.

Add the ingredients; gently stir to mix well.

Properly close the top lid; make sure that the safety valve is properly locked.

Press "MEAT/STEW" Cooking function; set pressure level to "HIGH" and set the Cooking time to 6 minutes.

Allow the pressure to build to cook the ingredients.

After Cooking time is over press "CANCEL" setting. Find and press "NPR" Cooking function. This setting is for the natural release of inside pressure, and it takes around 10 minutes to release pressure slowly.

Slowly open the lid, take out the cooked recipe in serving containers. Serve warm.

Nutrition:

Calories: 423

Protein: 36 g

Fat: 34 g

Carbohydrates: 14 g

Garlic Pulled Pork

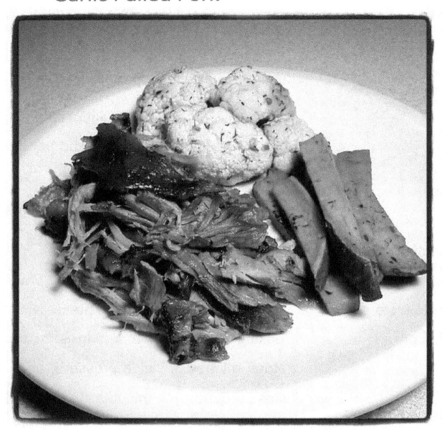

Preparation Time: *5 minutes*

Cooking Time: *1 hour and 40 minutes*

Servings: *12*

Ingredients:

- 4-pounds pork shoulder, boneless and cut into 3 pieces
- 2 tablespoons soy sauce
- 2 tablespoons brown sugar
- 1 cup chicken broth
- 10 cloves garlic, finely chopped

- 2 tablespoons butter, melted at room temperature

Directions:

In a mixing bowl, combine the broth, soy sauce, and brown sugar. Add the garlic and stir to combine.

Preheat your instant pot using the sauté setting and add the butter.

When warmed, add the pork pieces and stir-cook until browned on all sides.

Add the soy mix; stir gently.

Seal the lid and cook on high pressure for 90 minutes using the manual setting.

Let the pressure release naturally, about 10 minutes.

Uncover the instant pot; take out the meat and shred it using a fork.

Return the shredded meat to the instant pot and stir the mixture well.

Transfer to serving plates and serve.

Nutrition:

Calories: 142

Protein: 11.2 g

Fat: 8.2 g

Carbohydrates: 3.5 g

Buttered Pork Chops

Preparation Time: 15 minutes

Cooking Time: 15 minutes

Servings: 4

Ingredients:

- Pork Chops (4)
- Salt (1 t.)
- Bacon Grease (2 T.)
- Butter (4 T.)
- Pepper (1 t.)

Directions:

If you are looking for a quick and easy meal, look no further than buttered pork chops! Within twenty minutes, you'll be sitting down and enjoying your meal. You will want to start off this recipe by taking out your pork chops and seasoning them on either side. If you need more than a teaspoon of salt and pepper, feel free to season as desired.

Next, you are going to want to place your skillet over high heat and place the bacon grease and butter into the bottom.

Once the butter is melted and the grease is sizzling, pop the pork chops into the skillet and sear on either side for three to four minutes. In the end, the pork should be a nice golden color.

When the meat is cooked as desired, remove the skillet from the heat and enjoy your meal!

Nutrition:

Calories: 450

Fats: 30g

Proteins: 45g

Quick and Easy Pork Loin Roast

Preparation Time: 45 minutes

Cooking Time: 30 minutes

Servings: 6

Ingredients:

- Bacon Grease (1 T.)
- Salt (1 t.)
- Pork Loin (3 Lbs.)
- Pepper (1 t.)

Directions:

Even with just four ingredients, you will be surprised how delicious this recipe will be! Before you start cooking, you will want to go ahead and heat your oven to 375 degrees.

As the oven is warming up, take out your baking pan and gently place the pork loin into the bottom. Once in place, go ahead and rub the salt and pepper all over the sides. Be sure that each side is coated to help even out the flavor over the loin.

Finally, pop the dish into the oven for one hour. At the end of this time, the meat should be cooked through to your liking. Remember that you will want your meat to be slightly rare to get the most nutrients from it.

Remove the meat from the oven, allow it to cool for several minutes, and then your meat is ready to be enjoyed.

Nutrition:

Calories: 520

Fats: 35g

Protein: 50g

Cheese and Ham Roll-ups

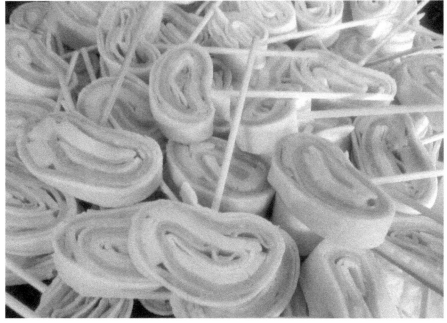

Preparation Time: 20 minutes

Cooking Time: 15 minutes

Servings: 7

Ingredients:

- Eggs (2)
- Ham, Diced (1 C.)
- Cheddar Cheese, Shredded (.50 C.)
- Mozzarella Cheese, Shredded (.75 C.)
- Parmesan Cheese (.50 C.)

Directions:

If you ever find yourself craving a snack while following the Carnivore Diet, this little recipe should do the trick! Start off by heating your oven to 375 degrees.

As the oven warms up, take out a mixing bowl and combine the egg and shredded cheeses together. Once the clumps are taken out, you can also add in the ham and give everything a good stir.

Now, you will want to take out a baking sheet and line it with parchment paper. When this is in place, divide your mixture onto the parchment paper for six or eight rolls.

When you are ready, place it into the oven and cook these for about twenty minutes. By the end, the cheese should create a brown crust.

If it looks like this, remove it from the oven, allow the roll-ups to cool, and enjoy your quick and easy snack!

Nutrition:

Calories: 200

Fats: 15g

Proteins: 15g

Meat Cup Snacks

Preparation Time: 25 minutes

Cooking Time: 15 minutes

Servings: 4

Ingredients:

- Eggs (6)
- Ham (6 Slices)
- Pepper (1 t.)
- Shredded Cheddar Cheese (.50 C.)

Directions:

Looking for another great snack? These will be perfect for breakfast, lunch, or dinner! Start off by heating the oven to 375 degrees. As it warms up, you can prep for this recipe by taking out a muffin tin and greasing it up with butter or bacon grease. If you want to avoid a mess, you can also use silicone muffin tins.

Once you are ready, take your slices of ham and line each hole with them, carefully placing them into a bottom.

When the ham is in place, get out a skillet and scramble the six eggs until they reach the desired consistency. Once cooked through, go ahead and scoop the scrambled egg into the muffin tin and place it on top of the ham.

For a final touch, sprinkle the egg with some shredded cheddar cheese. At this point, feel free to season these cups with salt and pepper. If not, they are going to taste delicious without any seasoning!

Finally, pop the muffin tin into your oven for about ten minutes. At the end of this time, the cheese should be melted and a nice golden color. If it looks like this, remove from the oven, allow to cool, and enjoy!

Nutrition:

Calories: 250

Fats: 15g

Proteins: 20g

Pork and Cheese Stuffed Peppers

Preparation Time: 30 minutes

Cooking Time: 25 minutes

Servings: 2

Ingredients:

- 2 sweet Italian peppers, deveined and halved
- 1/2 Spanish onion, finely chopped
- 1 cup marinara sauce
- 1/2 cup cheddar cheese, grated
- 4 ounces pork, ground

Directions:

Heat 1 tablespoon of canola oil in a saucepan over a moderate heat. Then, sauté the onion for 3 to 4 minutes until tender and fragrant.

Add in the ground pork; cook for 3 to 4 minutes more. Add in Italian seasoning mix. Spoon the mixture into the pepper halves.

Spoon the marinara sauce into a lightly greased baking dish. Arrange the stuffed peppers in the baking dish.

Bake in the preheated oven at 395 degrees F for 17 to 20 minutes. Top with cheddar cheese and continue to bake for about 5 minutes or until the top is golden brown. Bon appétit!

Nutrition:

313 Calories

21.3g Fat

5.7g Carbs

20.2g Protein

1.9g Fiber

Peppered Pork Rack

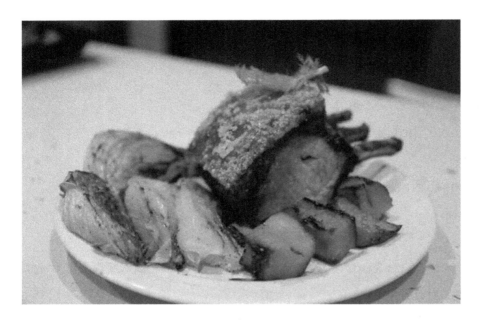

Preparation Time: 120 minutes

Cooking Time: 1 hour and 30 minutes

Servings: 6

Ingredients:

- Pepper (.25 C.)
- Pork Rib Rack (1)

Instructions:

While simple, this peppered pork rack can become a staple in your new carnivore diet because it is easy to make and delicious! You'll want to start off by heating your oven only to 375 degrees.

As the oven warms up, you will want to prepare your rib rack. Be sure that you coat the roast with the pepper seasoning. While a quarter of a cup of pepper may seem like a lot, you will want this much for maximum flavor.

When the meat is coated, place the roast into a baking dish, bones up. If you are ready to cook your meal, pop it into the oven for one hour and thirty minutes. Once it is cooked through, you can remove it from the oven and allow it to rest for around ten minutes.

Finally, cut the meat between the rib bones, and your meal is ready to be served!

Nutrition:

Calories: 400

Fats: 15g

Proteins: 30g

Pork Belly

Preparation Time: 30 minutes

Cooking Time: 1 hour and 30 minutes

Servings: 4

Ingredients:

Pork Belly (2 Lbs.)

Black Pepper (1 T.)

Butter (1 T.)

Directions:

As you can already tell, pork belly is high in fat and high in calories. The good news is that you are on the carnivore diet, and none of that matters; bring on the pork belly! To start off, you are going to want to heat your oven to 400 degrees.

To prepare your pork belly, you are going to want to score the belly skin. You will want to be careful not to cut the meat during this step, so take your time. When this is completed, go ahead and rub on the salt and pepper. You can use as much or as little seasoning as you desire!

When you are ready, place the pork belly into a roasting pan and place into the oven for thirty minutes. After this time has passed, you will want to turn the heat down to 320 degrees and then roast it for another twenty-five minutes per half-pound of meat.

Once the pork belly has cooked through, you have the option to switch on the broiler for a few minutes. By doing this, you can achieve a nice, crispy skin to dig into!

When your meat is cooked to the desired temperature, you will want to remove the dish from your oven carefully. I suggest waiting thirty minutes or so to allow the flavors to form in your pork belly fully. After that, you can slice up the meat, and your meal is ready to be served!

Nutrition:

Calories: 1,200

Fats: 120g

Proteins: 20g

Easy Pork Chops

Preparation Time: 10 minutes

Cooking Time: 20 or so minutes

Servings: 4

Ingredients:

- 4 pork chops, boneless
- 1 tablespoon extra-virgin olive oil
- 1 cup chicken stock, low-sodium
- A pinch of black pepper
- 1 teaspoon sweet paprika

Directions:

Heat up a pan while using the oil over medium-high heat, add pork chops, brown them for 5 minutes on either sides, add paprika, black pepper and stock, toss, cook for fifteen minutes more, divide between plates and serve by using a side salad.

Enjoy!

Nutrition:

Calories: 272

Fat: 4

Fiber: 8

Carbs: 14

Protein: 17

Coffee BBQ Pork Belly

Preparation Time: 20 minutes

Cooking Time: 50 minutes

Servings: 4

Ingredients:

- Beef stock (1.5 cups)
- Low-carb barbecue dry rub (as needed)
- Instant Espresso Powder (2 tbsp.)
- Pork belly (2 lb.)
- Olive oil (4 tbsp.)

Directions:

Set the oven at 350° F.

Warm the beef stock in a small saucepan using medium heat until hot - not boiling.

Mix in the dry barbecue rub and espresso powder until well combined.

Place the pork belly, skin side up in a shallow dish and drizzle half of the oil over the top, rubbing it over the entire pork belly.

Pour the hot stock around the pork belly and cover the dish tightly with aluminum foil. Bake it for 45 minutes.

Note: Slice into eight thick slices or 16 slices if you like a crispy pork belly.

Warm the remaining olive oil in a skillet using med-high heat and sear each slice for three minutes per side or until the desired level of crispiness is reached.

Nutrition:

Calories: 644

Protein: 24 g

Fat: Content: 68 g

Net Carbohydrates: 3 g

Mustard and Rosemary Pork Tenderloin

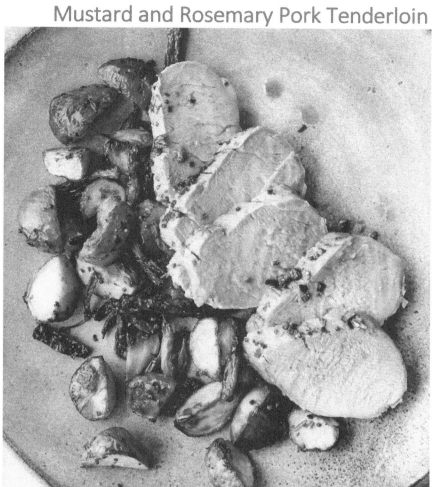

Preparation Time: 10 minutes

Cooking Time: 15 minutes plus 5 minutes resting time

Servings:4

Ingredients:

- ½ cup fresh parsley leaves
- ¼ cup dijon mustard

- 6 garlic cloves
- 3 tablespoons fresh rosemary leaves
- 3 tablespoons extra-virgin olive oil
- ½ teaspoon sea salt
- ¼ teaspoon freshly ground black pepper
- 1 (1½-pound) pork tenderloin

Directions:

Preheat the oven to 400°F.

In a blender or food processor, combine the parsley, mustard, garlic, rosemary, olive oil, salt, and pepper. Pulse in 1-second pulses, about 20 times, until a paste forms. Rub this paste all over the tenderloin and put the pork on a rimmed baking sheet.

Bake the pork for about 15 minutes, or until it registers 165°F on an instant-read meat thermometer.

Let rest for 5 minutes, slice, and serve.

Nutrition:

Calories: 362

Total Fat: 18g

Total Carbs: 5g

Sugar: <1g

Fiber: 2g

Protein: 2g

Sodium: 515m

Stuffed Pork Loin with Sun-Dried Tomato and Goat Cheese

Preparation Time: 15 minutes

Cooking Time: 40 minutes

Servings: 6

Ingredients:

- 1 to 1½ pounds pork tenderloin
- 1 cup crumbled goat cheese
- 4 ounces frozen spinach, thawed and well drained
- 2 tablespoons chopped sun-dried tomatoes
- 2 tablespoons extra-virgin olive oil (or seasoned oil marinade from sun-dried tomatoes), plus ¼ cup, divided
- ½ teaspoon salt
- ½ teaspoon freshly ground black pepper
- Zucchini Noodles or sautéed greens, for serving

Directions:

Preheat the oven to 350°F. Cut cooking twine into eight (6-inch) pieces.

Cut the pork tenderloin in half lengthwise, leaving about an inch border, being careful to not cut all the way through to the other side. Open the tenderloin like a book to form a large rectangle. Place it between two pieces of parchment paper or plastic wrap and pound to about ¼-inch thickness with a meat mallet, rolling pin, or the back of a heavy spoon.

In a small bowl, combine the goat cheese, spinach, sun-dried tomatoes, 2 tablespoons olive oil, salt, and pepper and mix to incorporate well.

Spread the filling over the surface of the pork, leaving a 1-inch border from one long edge and both short edges. To roll, start from the long edge with filling and roll towards the opposite edge. Tie cooking twine around the pork to secure it closed, evenly spacing each of the eight pieces of twine along the length of the roll.

In a Dutch oven or large oven-safe skillet, heat ¼ cup olive oil over medium-high heat. Add the pork and brown on all sides. Remove from the heat, cover, and bake until the pork is cooked through, 45 to 75 minutes, depending on the thickness of the pork. Remove from the oven and let rest for 10 minutes at room temperature.

To serve, remove the twine and discard. Slice the pork into medallions and serve over Zucchini Noodles or sautéed greens, spooning the cooking oil and any bits of filling that fell out during cooking over top.

Nutrition:

Calories: 270

Total Fat: 21g

Total Carbs: 2g

Net Carbs: 1g

Fiber: 1g

Protein: 20g

Sodium: 323mg

Flank Steak with Orange-Herb Pistou

Preparation Time: 10 minutes

Cooking Time: 20 minutes

Servings: 4

Ingredients:

- 1 pound flank steak
- 8 tablespoons extra-virgin olive oil, divided
- 2 teaspoons salt, divided
- 1 teaspoon freshly ground black pepper, divided
- ½ cup chopped fresh flat-leaf Italian parsley
- ¼ cup chopped fresh mint leaves
- 2 garlic cloves, roughly chopped
- Zest and juice of 1 orange or 2 clementines
- 1 teaspoon red pepper flakes (optional)
- 1 tablespoon red wine vinegar

Directions:

Heat the grill to medium-high heat or, if using an oven, preheat to 400°F.

Rub the steak with 2 tablespoons olive oil and sprinkle with 1 teaspoon salt and ½ teaspoon pepper. Let sit at room temperature while you make the pistou.

In a food processor, combine the parsley, mint, garlic, orange zest and juice, remaining 1 teaspoon salt, red pepper flakes (if using), and remaining ½ teaspoon pepper. Pulse until finely chopped. With the processor running, stream in the red wine vinegar and remaining 6 tablespoons olive oil until well combined. This pistou will be more oil-based than traditional basil pesto.

Cook the steak on the grill, 6 to 8 minutes per side. Remove from the grill and allow to rest for 10 minutes on a cutting board. If cooking in the oven, heat a large oven-safe skillet (cast iron works great) over high heat. Add the steak and seer, 1 to 2 minutes per side, until browned. Transfer the skillet to the oven and cook 10 to 12 minutes, or until the steak reaches your desired temperature.

To serve, slice the steak and drizzle with the pistou.

Nutrition:

Calories: 441

Total Fat: 36g

Total Carbs: 3g

Net Carbs: 3g

Fiber: 0g

Protein: 25g

Sodium: 1237mg

Beef Kofta

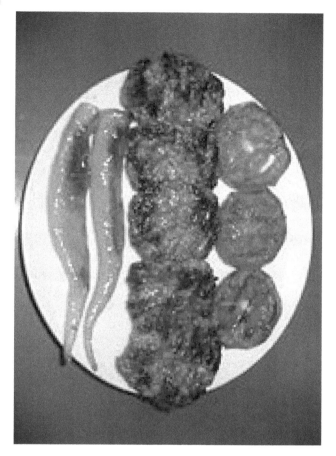

Preparation Time: 10 minutes

Cooking Time: 15 minutes

Servings: 4

Ingredients:

- 1 lb. ground beef
- 1/2 cup minced onions
- 1 tablespoon olive oil
- 1/2 teaspoon salt
- 1/2 teaspoon ground coriander

- 1/2 teaspoon ground cumin
- 1/4 teaspoon ground cinnamon
- 1/4 teaspoon allspice
- 1/4 teaspoon dried mint leaves

Directions:

Grab a large bowl and add all the ingredients.

Stir well to combine then use your hands to shape into ovals or balls.

Carefully thread onto skewers then brush with oil.

Pop into the grill and cook uncovered for 15 minutes, turning often.

Serve and enjoy.

Nutrition:

Calories: 216

Net carbs: 4g

Fat: 19g

Protein: 25g

Spicy Beef with Olives and Feta

Preparation Time: 3 hours

Cooking Time: 6 hours

Servings: 6-8

Ingredients:

- 2 lb. stewing beef, cut into ½" pieces
- 2 x 15 oz. cans chili-seasoned diced tomatoes, undrained
- 1 cup assorted olives, pitted and halved
- 1/2 teaspoon salt
- 1/4 teaspoon pepper
- 2 cups cooked basmati rice
- 1/2 cup crumbled feta cheese

Directions:

Open the lid of your slow cooker and add the beef, tomatoes and olives. Stir well.

Cover and cook on high for 5-6 hours or low for 8-9 ours until tender.

Season well then serve with the rice and feta cheese.

Serve and enjoy.

Nutrition:

Calories: 380

Net carbs: 14g

Fat: 19g

Protein: 36g

Best Ever Beef Stew

Preparation Time: 1 hour

Cooking Time: 2 hours

Servings: 6

Ingredients:

- 2 tablespoons olive oil
- 1 1/3 lb. extra- lean diced beef
- 1 large onion, sliced
- 1½ tablespoons chopped rosemary
- 5 garlic cloves, sliced
- 2/3 cup red wine (or extra stock)
- 1 2/3 cup beef stock
- 1 x 14 oz. can cherry tomatoes
- 3 mixed peppers, deseeded and thickly sliced
- 2 x 14 oz. can butterbeans, rinsed and drained
- 1 x 2.4 oz. pouch pitted Kalamata olives
- 2 tablespoons corn flour

Directions:

Preheat the oven to 280°F.

Place a Dutch oven over a medium heat and add 1 tablespoon oil.

Place the beef onto a flat surface, season well and cook in two batches.

Remove and place onto a plate when cooked.

Add the remaining oil and cook the onion, rosemary and garlic for 5 minutes until soft.

Add a pinch of salt then pour in the wine, scraping and browned bits from the pan.

Add the beef stock, tomatoes and peppers, stir well.

Add the beef, cover and bring to a simmer.

Pop into the oven and leave to cook for 2 hours.

Add the butterbeans and olive and pop back into the oven for 30 minutes.

Find a small bowl and combine the corn starch with a little water.

Pour gently into the stew, stir well and simmer until thickened.

Serve and enjoy.

Nutrition:

Calories: 337

Net carbs: 15g

Fat: 10g

Protein: 31g

One Pot Mediterranean Spiced Beef and Macaroni

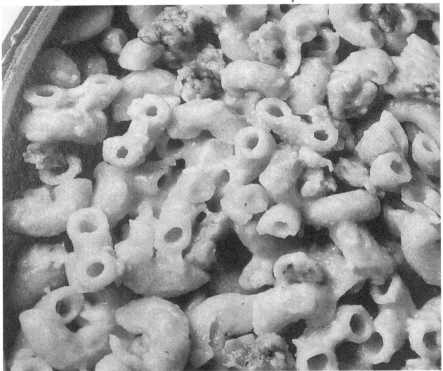

Preparation Time: 25 minutes

Cooking Time: 10 minutes

Servings: 4

Ingredients:

- 2 tablespoons olive oil
- 1 lb. ground beef
- 1 cup onion, diced
- 3 cloves garlic minced
- 1 teaspoon ground cinnamon
- ½ teaspoon kosher salt
- ¼ teaspoon cayenne pepper

- ¼ teaspoon ground cloves

- ½ cup red wine

- 2 Roma tomatoes diced

- 8 oz. can tomato sauce

- 2 cups macaroni or cavatappi noodles

- 2 cups beef broth

- ¼ cup parmesan cheese, grated

Directions:

Place a large pan over a medium heat and add the olive oil.

Add the beef, onion and garlic and cook for 10 minutes or so until soft.

Drain away the remaining grease then add the cinnamon, cayenne and cloves.

Cook for 3-4 minutes then add the red wine, tomatoes and tomato sauce.

Simmer for 5 minutes then add the noodles and the broth. Stir together.

Reduce the heat to low, cover and cook for 25 minutes until the noodles are cooked.

Top with parmesan and serve.

Nutrition:

Calories: 643

Net carbs: 57g

Fat: 23g

Protein: 35g

Beef and Cheese Gratin

Preparation Time: 5 minutes

Cooking Time: 15 minutes

Servings: 4

Ingredients:

- 1 ½ lb. steak mince
- 2/3 cup beef stock
- 3 oz. Mozzarella or cheddar cheese, grated
- 3 oz. butter, melted
- 7 oz. breadcrumbs
- 1 tablespoon extra-virgin olive oil
- 1 x roast vegetable pack
- 1 x red onion, diced
- 1 x red pepper, diced
- 1 x 14 oz. can chopped tomatoes
- 1 x zucchini, diced
- 3 cloves garlic, crushed
- 1 tablespoon Worcestershire sauce
- For the topping…
- Fresh thyme

Directions:

Pop a skillet over a medium heat and add the oil.

Add the red pepper, onion, zucchini and garlic. Cook for 5 minutes.

Add the beef and cook for five minutes.

Throw in the tinned tomatoes, beef stock and Worcestershire sauce then stir well.

Bring to the boil then simmer for 6 minutes.

Divide between the bowls and top with the thyme.

Serve and enjoy.

Nutrition:

Calories: 678

Net carbs: 24g

Fat: 45g

Protein: 48g

Beef Cacciatore

Preparation Time: 10 minutes

Cooking Time: 40 minutes

Servings: 5

Ingredients:

- 1 lb. beef, cut into thin slices
- 1/4 cup extra virgin olive oil
- 1 onion, chopped
- 2 red bell peppers, chopped
- 1 orange bell pepper, chopped
- Salt and pepper, to taste
- 1 cup tomato sauce

Directions:

Place a skillet over a medium heat and add the oil.

Add the meat and cook until browned.

Add the onions and peppers and cook for 3-5 minutes.

Throw in the tomato sauce, salt and pepper, stir well then bring to a simmer.

Cover and cook for 40 minutes until the meat is tender.

Pour off as much sauce as you can then whizz in a blender.

Pour back into the pan and heat again for 5 minutes.

Serve with pasta or rice and enjoy.

Nutrition:

Calories: 428

Net carbs: 16g

Fat: 35g

Protein: 12g

Greek Beef and Veggie Skewers

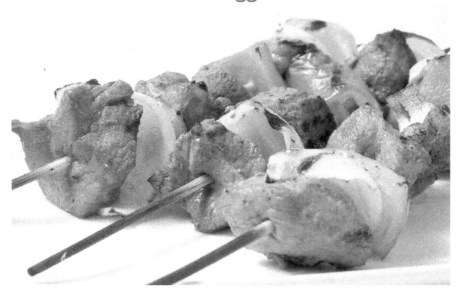

Preparation Time: 20 minutes

Cooking Time: 10 minutes

Servings: 6-8

Ingredients:

- For the beef skewers…
- 1 ½ lb. skirt steak, cut into cubes
- 1 teaspoon grated lemon zest
- ½ teaspoon coriander seeds, ground
- ½ teaspoon salt
- 2 garlic cloves, chopped
- 2 tablespoons olive oil
- 2 bell peppers, seeded and cubed
- 4 small green zucchinis, cubed
- 24 cherry tomatoes
- 2 tablespoons extra virgin olive oil

- To serve…
- Store-bought hummus
- 1 lemon, cut into wedges

Directions:

Grab a large bowl and add all the ingredients. Stir well.

Cover and pop into the fridge for at least 30 minutes, preferably overnight.

Preheat the grill to high and oil the grate.

Take a medium bowl and add the peppers, zucchini, tomatoes and oil. Season well

Just before cooking, start threading everything onto the skewers. Alternate veggies and meat as you wish.

Pop into the grill and cook for 5 minutes on each side.

Serve and enjoy.

Nutrition:

Calories: 938

Net carbs: 65g

Fat: 25g

Protein: 87g

Pork Tenderloin with Orzo

Preparation Time: 10 minutes

Cooking Time: 20 minutes

Servings: 6

Ingredients:

- 1-1/2 lb. pork tenderloin
- 1 teaspoon coarsely ground pepper
- 2 tablespoons extra virgin olive oil
- 3 quarts water
- 1 1/4 cups uncooked orzo pasta
- 1/4 teaspoon salt
- 6 oz. fresh baby spinach
- 1 cup grape tomatoes, halved
- 3/4 cup crumbled feta cheese

Directions:

Place the pork onto a flat surface and rub with the pepper.

Cut into the 1" cubes.

Place a skillet over a medium heat and add the oil.

Add the pork and cook for 10 minutes until no longer pink.

Fill a Dutch oven with water and place over a medium heat. Bring to a boil.

Stir in the orzo and cook uncovered for 8-10 minutes.

Stir through the spinach then drain.

Add the tomatoes to the pork, heat through then stir through orzo and cheese.

Serve and enjoy.

Nutrition:

Calories: 372

Net carbs: 34g

Fat: 11g

Protein: 31g

Grilled Pork Chops with Tomato Salad

Preparation Time: 15 minutes

Cooking Time: 15 minutes

Servings: 4

Ingredients:

- For the pork chops…
- 4 x 6 oz. boneless pork chops
- 1 tablespoon canola oil
- 1-2 tablespoons dry rub pork seasoning
- 1 teaspoon dried oregano
- For the tomato salad…
- 1 lb. medium size tomatoes, quartered
- 1 cup fresh Italian flat leaf parsley, leaves roughly chopped
- 1/3 cup sliced red onion
- 1/4 cup capers
- 1 clove garlic, pressed or minced
- 2 tablespoons extra virgin olive oil
- 1/2 lemon
- 1/2 teaspoon kosher salt
- 1/2 teaspoon freshly ground black pepper
- 1/2 cup feta cheese

Directions:

Preheat the grill to 350°F.

Brush the pork chops with oil and season well with the rub and oregano.

Leave to rest for 5-10 minutes as the grill warms.

Meanwhile, grab a large bowl and add the salad ingredients. Stir well and pop into the fridge until ready to be served.

Cook the pork chops for 10 minutes or so, turning halfway through.

Remove from the pan and leave to rest for five minutes before cutting.

Enjoy with the salad and chunks of feta.

Nutrition:

Calories: 340

Net carbs: 6g

Fat: 20g

Protein: 31g

Boneless Pork Chops with Summer Veggies

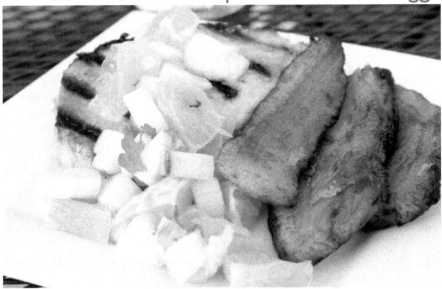

Preparation Time: 10 minutes

Cooking Time: 25 minutes

Servings: 4

Ingredients:

- 8 thin sliced center cut boneless pork chops
- 3/4 teaspoon Montreal chicken seasoning
- 1 small zucchini, julienned
- 1 small yellow squash, julienned
- 1 cup halved grape tomatoes
- 1 tablespoon extra-virgin olive oil
- Salt and pepper, to taste
- ¼ teaspoon oregano
- 3 cloves garlic, thinly sliced
- Extra virgin olive oil, to taste
- 1/4 cup pitted and sliced Kalamata olives
- 1/4 cup crumbled feta cheese
- Juice of ½ lemon

- 1 teaspoon grated lemon rind

Directions:

Preheat the oven to 450°F.

Grab a medium bowl and add the tomatoes, ½ tablespoon oil, 1/8 teaspoon salt, pepper and oregano. Stir well.

Place onto a baking sheet and pop into the oven for 10 minutes.

Add the sliced garlic and cook for 5 more minutes.

Remove from the oven and transfer to a large bowl.

Reduce the oven temperature to 200°F.

Place a large skillet over a medium heat, add ½ tablespoon olive oil, the zucchini and a pinch of salt and cook for 5 minutes until tender.

Transfer the zucchini to the bowl with the tomatoes and pop into the oven to keep warm.

Add more oil to the skillet and cook half the pork chops for about 2 minutes on each side.

Pop onto a platter then repeat with the second half. Pop onto a platter.

Remove the veggies from the oven then add the olives, lemon and lemon rind. Stir well to combine.

Top the pork with the veggies, top with feta then serve and enjoy.

Nutrition:

Calories: 230

Net carbs: 9g

Fat: 9g

Protein: 28g

One Skillet Mediterranean Pork and Rice

Preparation Time: 20 minutes

Cooking Time: 15 minutes

Servings: 4

Ingredients:

- 1/2 lb. roasted garlic & herb loin filet, cut in strips
- 2 tablespoons extra-virgin olive oil
- 2 carrots, chopped
- 1 bell pepper, chopped
- 1 onion, chopped
- 3 cloves garlic, minced
- 1/2 teaspoon oregano
- 2 cups vegetable stock
- 1 cup basmati rice
- 1/2 cup garbanzo beans
- 10 black pitted olives
- 1 lemon fresh parsley, chopped
- Salt and pepper, to taste

Directions:

Find a large skillet, add the oil and pop over a medium heat.

Add the pork and cook for five minutes until cooked through.

Transfer to a plate and pop to one side.

Add the carrots, bell pepper, onion and garlic and season well.

Cook for five minutes until the veggies are tender.

Add the rice and stir well.

Add the salt, pepper, oregano, lemon zest and stock.

Stir then bring to a boil.

Cover and simmer for 12-15 minutes until the rice is cooked.

Add the lemon juice and pork slices and stir well.

Add the garbanzo beans and olives and garnish with parsley.

Serve and enjoy.

Nutrition:

Calories: 341

Net carbs: 50g

Fat: 4g

Protein: 19g

Garlic and Rosemary Mediterranean Pork Roast

Preparation Time: 20 minutes

Cooking Time: 1 hour

Servings: 4

Ingredients:

- 2 - 2 ½ lb. pork sirloin roast
- 3 large garlic cloves, sliced
- Fresh rosemary, to taste
- 1 teaspoon salt
- 1/2 teaspoon pepper
- 2 tablespoons extra virgin olive oil

Directions:

Preheat the oven to 250°F.

Place the pork onto a flat surface and cut 1- deep slits into the top.

Place a sliver of garlic and a leaf of rosemary into each slit.

Season well with salt and pepper.

Place a skillet over a medium heat and add the olive oil.

Add the roast to the skillet and brown on all sides.

Grab a small roasting pan, add a rack to the inside and pop the roast on top.

Pop into the oven and cook for 1 hours until cooked, turning over halfway through cooking.

Remove from the oven, place onto a cutting board and tent with foil. Leave to rest for 15 minutes.

Serve and enjoy.

Nutrition:

Calories: 198

Net carbs: 8g

Fat: 32g

Protein: 22g

Pork Tenderloin with Roasted Vegetables

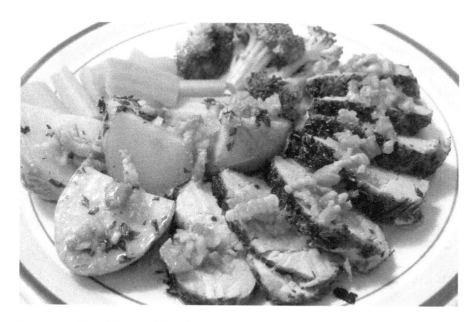

Preparation Time: 30 minutes

Cooking Time: 30 minutes

Servings: 8

Ingredients:

- 2 x 1 1/2 lb. pork tenderloins, halved crosswise
- 1 teaspoon ground coriander
- 1 teaspoon dried thyme
- 1 teaspoon granulated or powdered garlic
- 1 teaspoon coarse or kosher salt, plus extra to taste
- 1/2 teaspoon freshly ground black pepper, plus extra to taste
- 10 thyme sprigs
- 4 tablespoons olive oil
- 1 large red or yellow onion, peeled and cut into 1 ½" chunks
- 1 large fennel bulb., trimmed and cut into 1 ½" chunks

- 10 small white or red potatoes, chopped into chunks
- 2 jalapeno peppers, deseeded and sliced

Directions:

Preheat the oven to 425°F.

Find a small bowl and add the coriander, thyme, garlic, salt and pepper.

Stir well together then rub over the pork loins.

Pop a heavy skillet over a high heat and add about 2 tablespoons of olive oil.

Add the pork and sear on all sides.

Find a medium bowl and add the onions, fennel, potatoes, jalapenos and remaining oil.

Season well then toss to combine.

Place onto a rimmed baking sheet.

Top with the pork, tuck in thyme then pop into the oven for 30 minutes.

Remove the pork from the oven and place on a plate, covered to keep warm.

Spread the vegetables out over the tin and pop back into the oven for another 20 minutes until golden.

Slice the pork and serve with the roasted vegetables.

Serve and enjoy.

Nutrition:

Calories: 401

Net carbs: 40g

Fat: 12g

Protein: 34g

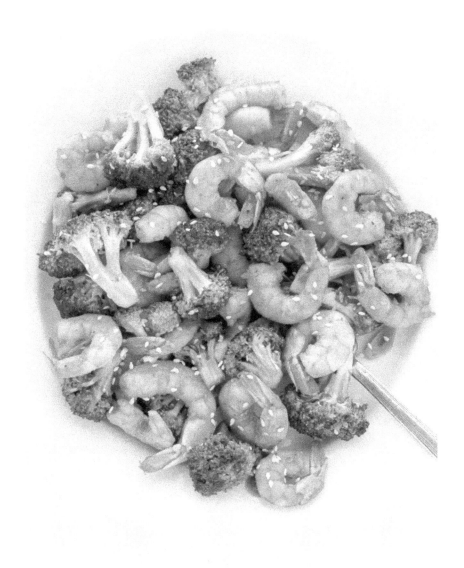

Crockpot Garlic and Shrimps

Preparation Time: 20 minutes

Cooking Time: 1 hour

Servings: 10

Ingredients:

- ¾ c. extra virgin olive oil
- 6 cloves of garlic, sliced
- 1 tsp. smoked Spanish paprika
- 1 tsp. salt
- ¼ tsp. black pepper
- ¼ tsp. red pepper flakes, crushed
- 2-pounds raw shrimp, shells removed and deveined
- 1 tbsp. parsley, minced

Directions:

Mix together olive oil, garlic, paprika, salt, pepper, and red pepper flakes.

Take the shrimp in the Crockpot and pour the spice mixture.

Stir to mix all ingredients.

Cook on low for 1 hour.

Garnish with parsley.

Nutrition:

Calories: 429

Carbohydrates: 1g

Protein: 18g

Fat: 24.5g

Roasted Red Snapper

Preparation Time: 5 minutes

Cooking Time: 45 minutes

Servings: 4

Ingredients:

- 1 (2 to 2½ pounds) whole red snapper, cleaned and scaled
- 2 lemons, sliced (about 10 slices)
- 3 cloves garlic, sliced
- 4 or 5 sprigs of thyme
- 3 tablespoons of cold salted butter, cut into small cubes, divided

Directions:

Preheat the oven to 350°F.

Cut a piece of foil to about the size of your baking sheet; put the foil on the baking sheet.

Make a horizontal slice through the belly of the fish to create a pocket.

Place 3 slices of lemon on the foil and the fish on top of the lemons.

Stuff the fish with the garlic, thyme, 3 lemon slices and butter. Reserve 3 pieces of butter.

Place the reserved 3 pieces of butter on top of the fish, and 3 or 4 slices of the lemon on top of the butter. Bring the foil together and seal it to make a pocket around the fish.

Put the fish in the oven and bake for 45 minutes. Serve with remaining fresh lemon slices.

Nutrition:

Carbohydrate – 12g

Protein - 54g

Fat – 13g

Calories: 345

Healthy Carrot & Shrimp

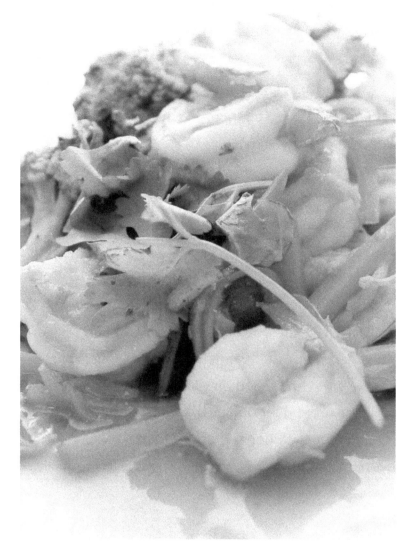

Preparation Time: 10 minutes

Cooking Time: 6 minutes

Serve: 4

Ingredients:

- 1 lb. shrimp, peeled and deveined

- 1 tbsp. chives, chopped
- 1 onion, chopped
- 1 tbsp. olive oil
- 1 cup fish stock
- 1 cup carrots, sliced
- Pepper
- Salt

Directions:

Add oil into the inner pot of instant pot and set the pot on sauté mode.

Add onion and sauté for 2 minutes.

Add shrimp and stir well.

Add remaining ingredients and stir well.

Cover the pot with lid and cook on high for 4 minutes.

Once done, release pressure using quick release. Remove lid.

Serve and enjoy.

Nutrition:

Calories 197

Fat 5.9 g

Carbohydrates 7 g

Sugar 2.5 g

Protein 27.7 g

Cholesterol 239 mg

Salmon with Potatoes

Preparation Time: 10 minutes

Cooking Time: 15 minutes

Serve: 4

Ingredients:

- 1 1/2 lbs. Salmon fillets, boneless and cubed
- 2 tbsp. olive oil
- 1 cup fish stock
- 2 tbsp. parsley, chopped
- 1 tsp. garlic, minced
- 1 lb. baby potatoes, halved
- Pepper
- Salt

Directions:

Add oil into the inner pot of instant pot and set the pot on sauté mode.

Add garlic and sauté for 2 minutes.

Add remaining ingredients and stir well.

Cover the pot with lid and cook on high for 13 minutes.

Once done, release pressure using quick release. Remove lid.

Serve and enjoy.

Nutrition:

Calories 362

Fat 18.1 g

Carbohydrates 14.5 g

Sugar 0 g

Protein 37.3 g

Cholesterol 76 mg

Honey Garlic Shrimp

Preparation Time: 10 minutes

Cooking Time: 5 minutes

Serve: 4

Ingredients:

- 1 lb. shrimp, peeled and deveined
- 1/4 cup honey
- 1 tbsp. garlic, minced
- 1 tbsp. ginger, minced
- 1 tbsp. olive oil
- 1/4 cup fish stock
- Pepper
- Salt

Directions:

Add shrimp into the large bowl. Add remaining ingredients over shrimp and toss well.

Transfer shrimp into the instant pot and stir well.

Cover the pot with lid and cook on high for 5 minutes.

Once done, release pressure using quick release. Remove lid.

Serve and enjoy.

Nutrition:

Calories 240

Fat 5.6 g

Carbohydrates 20.9 g

Sugar 17.5 g

Protein 26.5 g

Cholesterol 239 mg

Pan-Fried Cod

Preparation Time: 5 minutes

Cooking Time: 10 minutes

Servings: 4

Ingredients:

- ½ cup flour
- 1 teaspoon salt
- 1 teaspoon garlic powder
- 4 (4- to 5-ounce) cod fillets
- 3 tablespoons herb butter, either purchased or homemade (see recipe below)

Directions:

In a shallow plate combine the flour, salt, and garlic powder.

Mix the cod fillets in the seasoned flour until they are completely coated.

Preheat a medium pan over medium-high heat. Melt the herb butter.

Once the butter has melted, add the cod fillets to the pan and cook for 3 to 4 minutes on each side.

Remove from the pan and serve as part of a sandwich or with French fries.

Nutrition:

Carbohydrate – 12g

Protein - 27g

Fat – 10g

Calories: 248

Simple Lemon Clams

Preparation Time: 10 minutes

Cooking Time: 10 minutes

Serve: 4

Ingredients:

- 1 lb. clams, clean
- 1 tbsp. fresh lemon juice
- 1 lemon zest, grated
- 1 onion, chopped
- 1/2 cup fish stock
- Pepper
- Salt

Directions:

Add all ingredients into the inner pot of instant pot and stir well.

Cover the pot with lid and cook on high for 10 minutes.

Once done, release pressure using quick release. Remove lid.

Serve and enjoy.

Nutrition:

Calories 76

Fat 0.6 g

Carbohydrates 16.4 g

Sugar 5.4 g

Protein 1.8 g

Cholesterol 0 mg

Grilled Marinated Shrimp

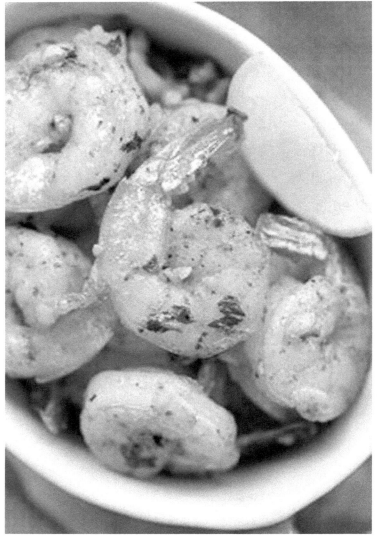

Preparation Time: 30 minutes

Cooking Time: 10 minutes

Servings: 6

Ingredients:

- 1 cup olive oil
- 1/4 cup chopped fresh parsley

- 1 lemon, juiced
- 2 tablespoons hot pepper sauce
- 3 cloves of garlic, finely chopped
- 1 tablespoon tomato puree
- 2 teaspoons dried oregano
- 1 teaspoon salt
- 1 teaspoon ground black pepper
- 2 pounds of shrimp, peeled

Directions:

Combine olive oil, parsley, lemon juice, hot sauce, garlic, tomato puree, oregano, salt, and black pepper in a bowl. Reserve a small amount for later. Pour the rest of the marinade into a large, resealable plastic bag with shrimp. Close and marinate in the fridge for 2 hours.

Preheat the grill on medium heat. Thread shrimp on skewers, poke once at the tail, and once at the head. Discard the marinade.

Lightly oil the grill. Cook the shrimp for 5 minutes on each side or until they are opaque, often baste with the reserved marinade.

Nutrition:

447 calories

37.5 grams of fat

3.7 grams of carbohydrates

25.3 g of protein

230 mg of cholesterol

800 mg of sodium

Grilled Salmon

Preparation Time: 15 minutes

Cooking Time: 16 minutes

Servings: 6

Ingredients:

- 1 1/2 pounds salmon fillet
- Pepper to taste
- Garlic powder to taste
- 1/3 cup soy sauce
- 1/3 cup of brown sugar
- 1/3 cup of water
- 1/4 cup vegetable oil

Directions:

Season the salmon fillets with lemon pepper, salt, and garlic powder.

Mix the soy sauce, brown sugar, water, and vegetable oil in a small bowl until the sugar is dissolved. Place the fish in a big resealable plastic bag with the soy sauce mixture, seal, and let marinate for at least 2 hours.

Preheat the grill on medium heat.

Lightly oil the grill. Place the salmon on the preheated grill and discard the marinade. Cook salmon 6 to 8 minutes per side or until the fish flakes easily with a fork.

Nutrition:

318 calories

20.1 grams of fat

13.2 g carbohydrates

20.5 g of protein

56 mg cholesterol

1092 mg of sodium

Cedar Planked Salmon

Preparation Time: 15 minutes

Cooking Time: 20 minutes

Servings: 6

Ingredients:

- 3 untreated cedar boards
- 1/3 cup of vegetable oil
- 1/3 cup soy sauce
- 1/4 cup chopped green onions
- 1 1/2 tablespoon rice vinegar
- 1 teaspoon sesame oil
- 1 teaspoon finely chopped garlic
- 1 tablespoon grated fresh ginger root
- 2 skinless salmon fillets

Directions:

Soak the cedar boards in hot water for at least 1 hour. Enjoy longer if you have time.

Combine vegetable oil, rice vinegar, sesame oil, soy sauce, green onions, ginger, and garlic in a shallow dish. Place the salmon fillets in the marinade and turn them over to coat them. Cover and marinate for a minimum of 15 minutes or a maximum of one hour.

Preheat an outside grill over medium heat. Place the shelves on the rack. The boards are ready when they start to smoke a little.

Place the salmon fillets on the shelves and discard the marinade — cover and grill for about 20 minutes. The fish is cooked if you can peel it with a fork.

Nutrition:

678 calories

45.8 g fat

1.7 g carbohydrates

61.3 g of protein

179 mg cholesterol

981 mg of sodium

Broiled Tilapia Parmesan

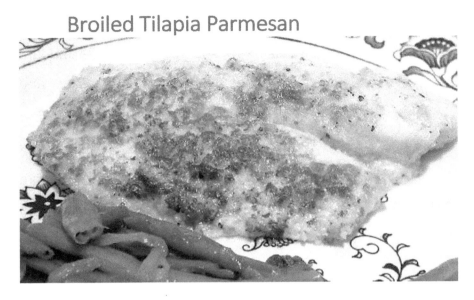

Preparation Time: 5 minutes

Cooking Time: 10 minutes

Servings: 8

Ingredients:

- 1/2 cup Parmesan cheese
- 1/4 cup butter, soft
- 3 tablespoons mayonnaise
- 2 tablespoons fresh lemon juice
- 1/4 teaspoon dried basil
- 1/4 teaspoon ground black pepper
- 1/8 teaspoon onion powder
- 1/8 teaspoon celery salt
- 2 pounds Tilapia fillets

Directions:

Preheat the grill on your oven. Grease a drip tray or grill pan with aluminum foil.

Combine parmesan, butter, mayonnaise, and lemon juice in a small bowl. Season with dried basil, pepper, onion powder, and celerysalt mixed well and set aside.

Place the fillets in a single layer on the prepared dish. Grill a few centimeters from the heat for 2 to 3 minutes, turn the fillets and grill for a few minutes. Remove the fillets from the oven and cover with the Parmesan cheese mixture on top. Grill for another 2 minutes or until the garnish is golden brown and fish flakes easily with a fork. Be careful not to overcook the fish.

Nutrition:

224 calories

12.8 g of fat

0.8 g carbohydrates

25.4 g of protein

63 mg cholesterol

220 mg of sodium.

Fish Tacos

Preparation Time: 40 minutes

Cooking Time: 15 minutes

Servings: 8

Ingredients:

- 1 cup flour
- 2 tablespoons corn flour
- 1 teaspoon baking powder
- 1/2 teaspoon of salt
- 1 egg
- 1 cup of beer
- 1/2 cup of yogurt
- 1/2 cup of mayonnaise
- 1 lime, juice
- 1 jalapeño pepper, minced
- 1 c. Finely chopped capers
- 1/2 teaspoon dried oregano
- 1/2 teaspoon ground cumin
- 1/2 teaspoon dried dill
- 1 teaspoon ground cayenne pepper
- 1 liter of oil for frying
- 1 pound of cod fillets, 2-3 ounces each
- 8 corn tortillas
- 1/2 medium cabbage, finely shredded

Directions:

Prepare beer dough: combine flour, corn flour, baking powder and salt in a large bowl. Mix the egg and the beer and stir in the flour mixture quickly.

To make a white sauce: combine yogurt and mayonnaise in a medium bowl. Gradually add fresh lime juice until it is slightly fluid — season with jalapeño, capers, oregano, cumin, dill, and cayenne pepper.

Heat the oil in a frying pan.

Lightly sprinkle the fish with flour. Dip it in the beer batter and fry until crispy and golden brown. Drain on kitchen paper. Heat the tortillas. Place the fried fish in a tortilla and garnish with grated cabbage and white sauce.

Nutrition:

409 calories

18.8 g of fat

43 grams of carbohydrates

17.3 g of protein

54 mg cholesterol

407 mg of sodium.

Grilled Tilapia with Mango Salsa

Preparation Time: 45 minutes

Cooking Time: 10 minutes

Servings: 2

Ingredients:

- 1/3 cup extra virgin olive oil
- 1 tablespoon lemon juice
- 1 tablespoon chopped fresh parsley
- 1 clove of garlic, minced
- 1 teaspoon dried basil
- 1 teaspoon ground black pepper
- 1/2 teaspoon salt
- 2 tilapia fillets (1 oz. each)
- 1 large ripe mango, peeled, pitted and diced
- 1/2 red pepper, diced
- 2 tablespoons chopped red onion
- 1 tablespoon chopped fresh coriander
- 1 jalapeño pepper, seeded and minced
- 2 tablespoons lime juice
- 1 tablespoon lemon juice
- salt and pepper to taste

Directions:

Mix extra virgin olive oil, 1 tablespoon lemon juice, parsley, garlic, basil, 1 teaspoon pepper, and 1/2 teaspoon salt in a bowl, then pour into a resealable plastic bag. Add the tilapia fillets, cover with the marinade, remove excess air, and close the bag. Marinate in the fridge for 1 hour.

Prepare the mango salsa by combining the mango, red pepper, red onion, coriander, and jalapeño pepper in a bowl. Add the lime juice and 1 tablespoon lemon juice and mix well. Season with salt and pepper and keep until serving.

Preheat a grill over medium heat and lightly oil.

Remove the tilapia from the marinade and remove the excess. Discard the rest of the marinade. Grill the fillets until the fish is no longer translucent in the middle and flake easily with the fork for 3 to 4 minutes on each side, depending on the thickness of the fillets. Serve the tilapia topped with mango salsa.

Nutrition:

634 calories

40.2 grams of fat

33.4 g carbohydrates

36.3 g of protein

62 mg cholesterol

697 mg of sodium.

Blackened Salmon Fillets

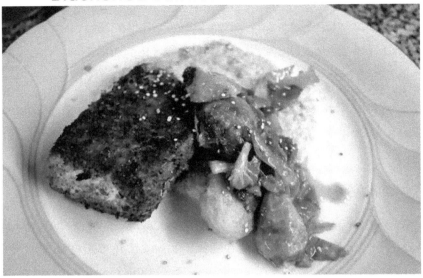

Preparation Time: 15 minutes

Cooking Time: 10 minutes

Servings: 4

Ingredients:

- 2 tablespoons paprika powder
- 1 tablespoon cayenne pepper powder
- 1 tablespoon onion powder
- 2 teaspoons salt
- 1/2 teaspoon ground white pepper
- 1/2 teaspoon ground black pepper
- 1/4 teaspoon dried thyme
- 1/4 teaspoon dried basil
- 1/4 teaspoon dried oregano
- 4 salmon fillets, skin and bones removed

- 1/2 cup unsalted butter, melted

Directions:

Combine bell pepper, cayenne pepper, onion powder, salt, white pepper, black pepper, thyme, basil and oregano in a small bowl.

Brush salmon fillets with 1/4 cup butter and sprinkle evenly with the cayenne pepper mixture. Sprinkle each fillet with ½ of the remaining butter.

Cook the salmon in a large heavy-bottomed pan, until dark, 2 to 5 minutes. Turn the fillets, sprinkle with the remaining butter and continue to cook until the fish easily peels with a fork.

Nutrition:

511 calories

38.3 grams of fat

4.5 grams of carbohydrates

37.4 g of protein

166 mg cholesterol

1248 mg of sodium

Seafood Enchiladas

Preparation Time: 15 minutes

Cooking Time: 30 minutes

Servings: 6

Ingredients:

- 1 onion, minced
- 1 tablespoon butter
- 1/2 pound of fresh crab meat
- 1/4 pound shrimp - peeled, gutted and coarsely chopped
- 8 grams of Colb.y cheese
- 6 flour tortillas (10 inches)
- 1 cup half and half cream
- 1/2 cup sour cream
- 1/4 cup melted butter
- 1 1/2 teaspoon dried parsley
- 1/2 teaspoon garlic salt

Directions:

Preheat the oven to 175 ° C (350 ° F).

Fry the onions in a large frying pan in 1 tablespoon butter until they are transparent. Remove the pan from the heat and stir in the crab meat and shrimp. Grate the cheese and mix half of the seafood.

Place a large spoon of the mixture in each tortilla. Roll the tortillas around the mixture and place them in a 9 x 13-inch baking dish.

In a saucepan over medium heat, combine half and half, sour cream, 1/4 cup butter, parsley and garlic salt. Stir until the mixture is lukewarm and mixed. Pour the sauce over the enchiladas and sprinkle with the remaining cheese.

Bake in the preheated oven for 30 minutes.

Nutrition:

607 calories

36.5 grams of fat

42.6 g carbohydrates

26.8 g of protein

136 mg of cholesterol

1078 mg of sodium.

Seafood Stuffing

Preparation Time: 25 minutes

Cooking Time: 30 minutes

Servings: 8

Ingredients:

- 1/2 cup butter
- 1/2 cup chopped green pepper
- 1/2 cup chopped onion
- 1/2 cup chopped celery
- Drained and flaky crabmeat
- 1/2 pound of medium-sized shrimp - peeled and deveined
- 1/2 cup spiced and seasoned breadcrumbs
- 1 mixture of filling for cornbread
- 2 tablespoons of white sugar, divided
- 1 can of mushroom soup (10.75 ounces) condensed
- 14.5 oz. chicken broth

Directions:

Melt the butter in a large frying pan over medium heat. Add pepper, onion, celery crabmeat and shrimp; boil and stir for about 5 minutes. Set aside.

In a large bowl, mix stuffing, breadcrumbs, and 1 tablespoon sugar. Stir the vegetables and seafood from the pan. Add the mushroom cream and as much chicken broth as you want. Pour into a 9 x 13-inch baking dish.

Bake in the preheated oven for 30 minutes or until lightly roasted.

Nutrition:

344 calories

15.7 grams of fat

28.4 g of carbohydrates22 g of protein

94 mg of cholesterol

1141 mg of sodium.

Scrumptious Salmon Cakes

Preparation Time: 15 minutes

Cooking Time: 15 minutes

Servings: 8

Ingredients:

- 2 cans of salmon, drained and crumbled
- 3/4 cup Italian breadcrumbs
- 1/2 cup chopped fresh parsley
- 2 eggs, beaten
- 2 green onions, minced
- 2 teaspoons seafood herbs
- 1 1/2 teaspoon ground black pepper
- 1 1/2 teaspoons garlic powder
- 3 tablespoons Worcestershire sauce
- 2 tablespoons Dijon mustard
- 3 tablespoons grated Parmesan
- 2 tablespoons creamy vinaigrette
- 1 tablespoon olive oil

Directions:

Combine salmon, breadcrumbs, parsley, eggs, green onions, seafood herbs, black pepper, garlic powder, Worcestershire sauce, parmesan cheese, Dijon mustard, and creamy vinaigrette; divide and shape into eight patties.

Heat olive oil in a large frying pan over medium heat. Bake the salmon patties in portions until golden brown, 5 to 7 minutes per side. Repeat if necessary with more olive oil.

Nutrition:

263 calories

12.3 g fat

10.8 g of carbohydrates

27.8 g of protein

95 mg cholesterol

782 mg of sodium

Easy Tuna Patties

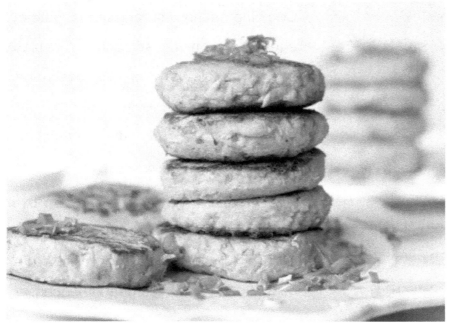

Preparation Time: 15 minutes

Cooking Time: 10 minutes

Servings: 4

Ingredients:

- 2 teaspoons lemon juice
- 3 tablespoons grated Parmesan
- 2 eggs
- 10 tablespoons Italian breadcrumbs
- 3 tuna cans, drained
- 3 tablespoons diced onion
- 1 pinch of ground black pepper
- 3 tablespoons vegetable oil

Directions:

Beat the eggs and lemon juice in a bowl. Stir in the Parmesan cheese and breadcrumbs to obtain a paste. Add tuna and onion until everything is well mixed. Season with black pepper. Form the tuna mixture into eight 1-inch-thick patties.

Heat the vegetable oil in a frying pan over medium heat; fry the patties until golden brown, about 5 minutes on each side.

Nutrition:

325 calories

15.5 grams of fat

13.9 g of carbohydrates

31.3 g of protein

125 mg cholesterol

409 mg of sodium

Heather's Grilled Salmon

Preparation Time: 10 minutes

Cooking Time: 10 minutes

Servings: 4

Ingredients:

- 1/4 cup brown sugar
- 1/4 cup olive oil
- 1/4 cup soy sauce
- 2 teaspoons lemon pepper
- 1 teaspoon dried thyme
- 1 teaspoon dried basil
- 1 teaspoon dried parsley
- 1/2 teaspoon garlic powder
- 4 (6 oz.) salmon fillets

Directions:

Whisk together the brown sugar, olive oil, soy sauce, lemon pepper, thyme, basil, parsley, and garlic powder in a bowl and pour into a resealable plastic bag.

Add the salmon fillets, coat with the marinade, squeeze out excess air, and seal the bag. Marinate in the refrigerator for at least 1 hour, turning occasionally.

Preheat an outdoor grill for medium heat, and lightly oil the grate. Remove the salmon from the marinade and shake off excess. Discard the remaining marinade.

Grill the salmon on the preheated grill until browned and the fish flakes easily with a fork, about 5 minutes on each side.

Nutrition:

380 calories

19.4 g fat

15.7 g carbohydrates

34.7 g protein

88 mg cholesterol

1251 mg sodium

Brown Butter Perch

Preparation Time: 15 minutes

Cooking Time: 10 minutes

Servings: 4

Ingredients:

- 1 cup flour
- 1 teaspoon salt
- 1/2 teaspoon finely ground black pepper
- 1/2 teaspoon cayenne pepper
- 8 oz. fresh perch fillets
- 2 tablespoons butter
- 1 lemon cut in half

Directions:

In a bowl, beat flour, salt, black pepper, and cayenne pepper. Gently squeeze the perch fillets into the flour mixture to coat well and remove excess flour.

Heat the butter in a frying pan over medium heat until it is foamy and brown hazel. Place the fillets in portions in the pan and cook them light brown, about 2 minutes on each side. Place the cooked fillets on a plate, squeeze the lemon juice, and serve.

Nutrition:

271 calories

11.5 g of fat

30.9 g of carbohydrates

12.6 g of protein

43 mg of cholesterol

703 mg of sodium.

Add the rice, salt, and 1 cup of the broth to the skillet. Stir the ingredients together and cook over low heat until most of the liquid is absorbed. Repeat steps with broth, adding ½ cup of broth at a time, and cook until all but ½ cup of the broth is absorbed.

Add the shrimp and scallops when you stir in the final ½ cup of broth. Cover and let cook for 10 minutes. Serve warm.

Nutrition:

Carbohydrate – 64g

Protein - 24g

Fat – 12g

Calories: 460

Appetizers

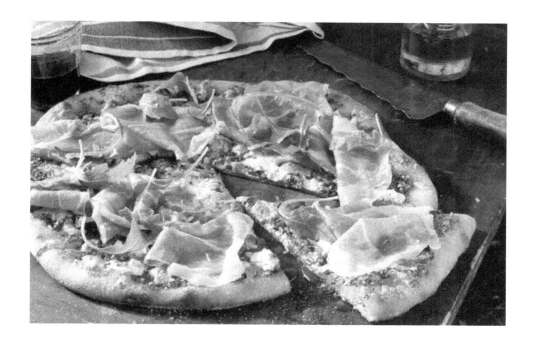

Greek Yogurt (Used as Dip)

Preparation time: 5 minutes

Cooking time: 0 minutes

Servings: 1

Ingredients:

- 6 oz Greek yogurt (plain and fat-free kind)

- ¼ cup crumbled tomato-basil feta cheese

- 2 tbsp Reduced-fat mayonnaise

- 2tbsp chopped fresh parsley

- Assorted fresh vegetables

Directions:

1. Mix yogurt, cheese, mayonnaise, and parsley in a small bowl. Divide the dip among bowls and serve with your favorite vegetables.

Nutrition:

Calories: 50

Carbs: 4g

Fat: 4g

Protein: 2g

Lemon Garlic Sesame Hummus Dip

Preparation time: 5 minutes

Cooking time: 0 minutes

Servings: 1

Ingredients:

- Tahini, lemon juice (fresh squeezed)
- 2 tbsp Extra virgin olive oil
- 2 tbsp toasted white sesame seeds
- 3 peeled and crushed garlic cloves
- 15 ounces drained garbanzo beans (reserve liquid)
- 1 ½ tbsp. minced lemon peel
- 1 tbsp. minced orange peel
- Sea salt
- White pepper

Directions:

1. Combine sesame seeds, extra virgin olive oil, garlic, garbanzo beans (reserve 1 tablespoon for garnish), lemon juice, and tahini in a food processor.

2. Keep adding the garbanzo bean liquid only if it is necessary until desired consistency.

3. Season hummus with sea salt and pepper and garnish with the reserved beans, and sprinkle with lemon and orange peel. Refrigerate until chilled.

Nutrition:

Calories: 60

Carbs: 6g

Fat: 3g

Protein: 2g

Creamy Greek Yogurt and Cucumber

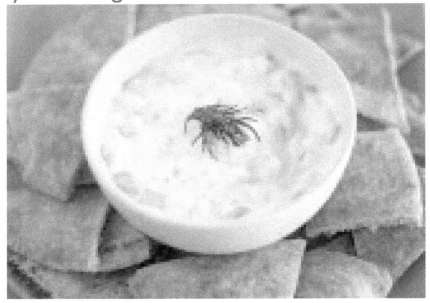

Preparation time: 5 minutes

Cooking time: 0 minutes

Servings: 1

Ingredients:

- 2 English cucumbers, thinly sliced
- Small bunch dill
- 1 ½ cups low-fat Greek yogurt
- 2 tbsp Fresh lemon juice
- 1 ½ tsp. mustard seeds
- Coarse salt and ground pepper

Directions:

1. Combine all your fixings in a bowl until combined well and dig in!

Nutrition:

Calories: 21

Carbs: 2g

Fat: 0g

Protein: 23g

Nachos

Preparation time: 5 minutes

Cooking time: 10 minutes

Servings: 4

Ingredients:

- 4-ounce restaurant-style corn tortilla chips
- 1 medium green onion, thinly sliced (about 1 tbsp.)
- 1 (4 ounces) package finely crumbled feta cheese
- 1 finely chopped and drained plum tomato
- 2 tbsp Sun-dried tomatoes in oil, finely chopped
- 2 tbsp Kalamata olives

Directions:

1. Mix an onion, plum tomato, oil, sun-dried tomatoes, and olives in a small bowl.
2. Arrange the tortillas chips on a microwavable plate in a single layer topped evenly with cheese—microwave on high for one minute.
3. Rotate the plate half turn and continue microwaving until the cheese is bubbly. Spread the tomato mixture over the chips and cheese and enjoy.

Nutrition:

Calories: 140

Carbs: 19g

Fat: 7g

Protein: 2g

Stuffed Celery

Preparation time: 15 minutes

Cooking time: 20 minutes

Servings: 3

Ingredients:

- Olive oil
- 1 clove garlic, minced
- 2 tbsp Pine nuts
- 2 tbsp dry-roasted sunflower seeds
- ¼ cup Italian cheese blend, shredded
- 8 stalks celery leaves
- 1 (8-ounce) fat-free cream cheese
- Cooking spray

Directions:

1. Sauté garlic and pine nuts over a medium setting for the heat until the nuts are golden brown. Cut off the wide base and tops from celery.
2. Remove two thin strips from the round side of the celery to create a flat surface.
3. Mix Italian cheese and cream cheese in a bowl and spread into cut celery stalks.
4. Sprinkle half of the celery pieces with sunflower seeds and a half with the pine nut mixture. Cover mixture and let stand for at least 4 hours before eating.

Nutrition:

Calories: 64

Carbs: 2g

Fat: 6g

Protein: 1g

Butternut Squash Fries

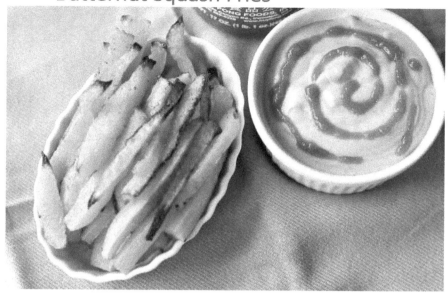

Preparation time: 5 minutes

Cooking time: 10 minutes

Servings: 2

Ingredients:

- 1 Butternut squash

- 1 tbsp Extra virgin olive oil

- ½ tbsp Grapeseed oil

- 1/8 tsp Sea salt

Directions:

1. Remove seeds from the squash and cut into thin slices. Coat with extra virgin olive oil and grapeseed oil. Add a sprinkle of salt and toss to coat well.

2. Arrange the squash slices onto three baking sheets and bake for 10 minutes until crispy.

Nutrition:

Calories: 40

Carbs: 10g

Fat: 0g

Protein: 1g

Dried Fig Tapenade

Preparation time: 5 minutes

Cooking time: 0 minutes

Servings: 1

Ingredients:

- 1 cup Dried figs
- 1 cup Kalamata olives
- ½ cup Water
- 1 tbsp Chopped fresh thyme
- 1 tbsp extra virgin olive oil
- ½ tsp Balsamic vinegar

Directions:

1. Prepare figs in a food processor until well chopped, add water, and continue processing to form a paste.

2. Add olives and pulse until well blended. Add thyme, vinegar, and extra virgin olive oil and pulse until very smooth. Best served with crackers of your choice.

Nutrition:

Calories: 249

Carbs: 64g

Fat: 1g

Protein: 3g

Speedy Sweet Potato Chips

Preparation time: 15 minutes

Cooking time: 60 minutes

Servings: 4

Ingredients:

- 1 large Sweet potato
- 1 tbsp Extra virgin olive oil
- Salt

Directions:

1. 300°F preheated oven. Slice your potato into nice, thin slices that resemble fries.

2. Toss the potato slices with salt and extra virgin olive oil in a bowl. Bake for about one hour, flipping every 15 minutes until crispy and browned.

Nutrition:

Calories: 150

Carbs: 16g

Fat: 9g

Protein: 1g

Nachos with Hummus (Mediterranean Inspired)

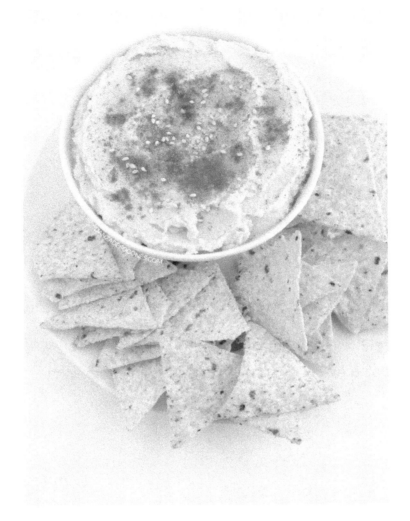

Preparation time: 15 minutes

Cooking time: 20 minutes

Servings: 4

Ingredients:

- 4 cups salted pita chips

- 1 (8 oz.) red pepper (roasted)

- Hummus

- 1 tsp Finely shredded lemon peel

- ¼ cup Chopped pitted Kalamata olives

- ¼ cup crumbled feta cheese

- 1 plum (Roma) tomato, seeded, chopped

- ½ cup chopped cucumber

- 1 tsp Chopped fresh oregano leaves

Directions:

1. 400°F preheated oven. Arrange the pita chips on a heatproof platter and drizzle with hummus.

2. Top with olives, tomato, cucumber, and cheese and bake until warmed through. Sprinkle lemon zest and oregano and enjoy while it's hot.

Nutrition:

Calories: 130

Carbs: 18g

Fat: 5g

Protein: 4g

Pineapple Mediterranean Dip

Preparation time: 5 minutes

Cooking time: 0 minutes

Servings: 1

Ingredients:

- 16 strawberries
- 8 bunches grapes
- 2 nectarines, thinly sliced
- 1 can pineapple (drained)
- Flaked and toasted coconut (¼ cup)
- Choc chip cookies

Directions:

1. Mix a pineapple, coconut, and yogurt in a bowl and top with fruit and cookies. Cover and refrigerate for one hour before eating.

Nutrition:

Calories: 100

Carbs: 0g

Fat: 2g

Protein: 2g

Mediterranean Inspired Tapenade

Preparation time: 5 minutes

Cooking time: 0 minutes

Servings: 1

Ingredients:

- 1 cup Pitted Kalamata olives
- 5 cloves garlic
- One lemon, juiced
- 2 tbsp Extra virgin olive oil
- 1 tbsp capers
- ½ tsp Allspice
- ¼ cup Chopped parsley

Directions:

1. Process all fixings using a food processor until blended well. Serve and enjoy!

Nutrition:

Calories: 80

Carbs: 2g

Fat: 7g

Protein: 0g

Hummus and Olive Pita Bread

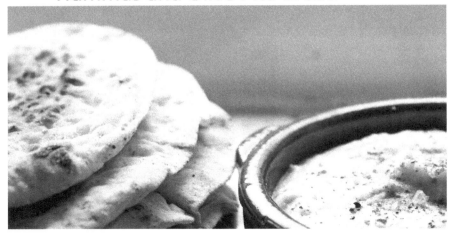

Preparation time: 5 minutes

Cooking time: 0 minutes

Servings: 3

Ingredients:

- 7 pita bread cut into 6 wedges each
- 1 (7 ounces) container plain hummus
- 1 tbsp Greek vinaigrette
- ½ cup Chopped pitted Kalamata olives

Directions:

1. Spread the hummus on a serving plate—Mix vinaigrette and olives in a bowl and spoon over the hummus. Enjoy with wedges of pita bread.

Nutrition:

Calories: 225

Carbs: 40g

Fat: 5g

Protein: 9g

Lime Yogurt Dip

Preparation time: 10 minutes

Cooking time: 0 minutes

Servings:4

Ingredients:

- 1 large cucumber, trimmed
- 3 oz Greek yogurt
- 1 teaspoon olive oil
- 3 tablespoons fresh dill, chopped
- 1 tablespoon lime juice
- 3/4 teaspoon salt
- 1 garlic clove, minced

Directions:

1. Shred the cucumber, then squeeze its juice. Then place the squeezed cucumber in the bowl.

2. Add Greek yogurt, olive oil, dill, lime juice, salt, and minced garlic. Mix up the mixture until homogenous—store it in the fridge for up to 2 days.

Nutrition:

Calories 44

Fat 1.8

Fiber 0.7

Carbs 5.1

Protein 3.2

Chicken Kale Wraps

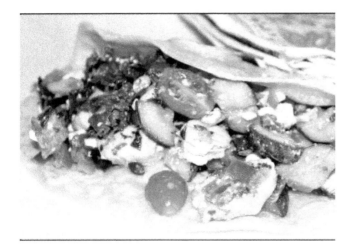

Preparation time: 10 minutes

Cooking time: 10 minutes

Servings:4

Ingredients:

- 4 kale leaves
- 4 oz chicken fillet
- ½ apple
- 1 tablespoon butter
- ¼ teaspoon chili pepper
- ¾ teaspoon salt
- 1 tablespoon lemon juice
- ¾ teaspoon dried thyme

Directions:

1. Chop the chicken fillet into small cubes. Then mix up the chicken with chili pepper and salt.

2. Heat butter in the skillet. Add chicken cubes. Roast them for 4 minutes.

3. Meanwhile, chop the apple into small cubes and add to the chicken. Mix up well.

4. Sprinkle the ingredients with lemon juice and dried thyme. Cook them for 5 minutes over medium-high heat.

5. Fill the kale leaves with the hot chicken mixture and wrap.

Nutrition:

Calories 106

Fat 5.1

Fiber 1.1

Carbs 6.3

Protein 9

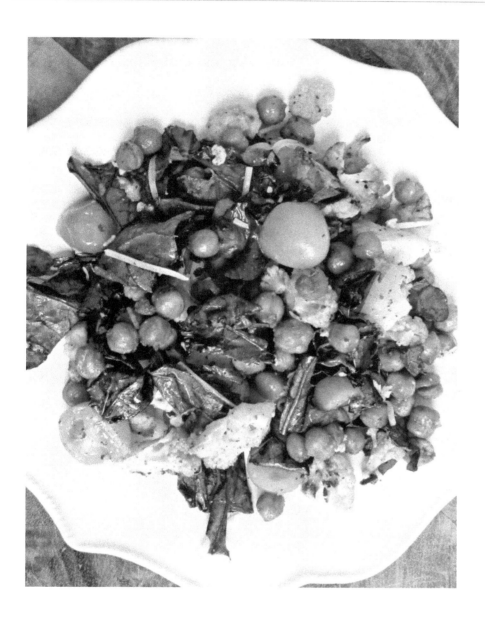

Italian Style Roasted Vegetables

Preparation Time: 15 minutes

Cooking Time: 30 minutes

Servings: 6

Ingredients:

- 8 ounces of mushrooms, baby Bella – clean and trim the ends
- 12 ounces of potatoes, baby – scrub and cube
- 12 ounces of tomatoes, Campari or cherry
- 2 zucchini sliced in 1" cubes – you can sub summer squash
- 10 to 12 peeled garlic cloves, large
- Oil, olive
- 1/2 tbsp. of oregano, dried
- 1 tsp. of thyme, dried
- Salt, kosher
- Pepper, ground
- Optional, to serve: Parmesan cheese, grated
- Optional: crushed pepper flakes, red

Directions:

Preheat oven to 425F.

Place veggies, garlic and mushrooms in large bowl. Generously drizzle with oil. Add thyme, oregano, kosher salt & ground pepper. Toss, combining well.

Spread potatoes only on oiled cookie sheet. Roast at 425F for 10 minutes. Add mushrooms and the rest of your veggies. Return to the oven and roast for 20 more minutes till vegetables become fork-tender. If they char a little, that's fine.

Lastly, sprinkle with Parmesan cheese and pepper flakes, if desired. Serve promptly.

Nutrition:

Calories: 86

Protein: 3.2g

Fat: 2.6g

Carbs: 14.2g

Mediterranean Diet Lemon Kale

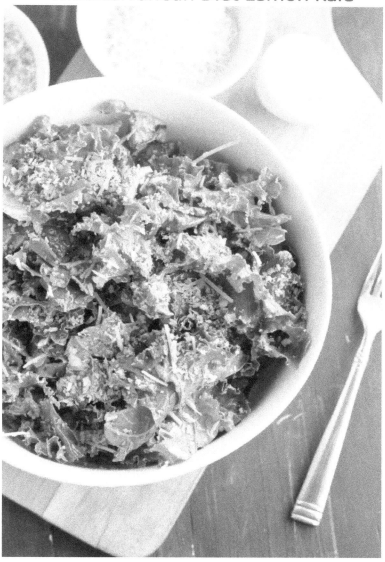

Preparation Time: 10 minutes

Cooking Time: 20 minutes

Servings: 6

Ingredients:

- 12 cups of kale, chopped

- 2 tbsp. of lemon juice, fresh if available
- 1 tbsp. of oil, olive +/- as you need it
- 1 tbsp. of garlic, minced
- 1 tsp. of soy sauce, low sodium
- Salt, kosher, as desired
- Pepper, ground, as desired

Directions:

Place steamer-type insert into pan. Fill with filtered water till just below bottom of steamer.

Cover pan. Bring water to boil on high heat. Then add the kale and put lid back on. Steam kale till barely tender, 7-10 minutes or so.

Whisk lemon juice, oil and garlic sauce together in large-sized bowl. Season as desired. Toss the steamed kale in dressing and coat well. Serve.

Nutrition:

Calories: 89

Protein: 4.6g

Fat: 3.2g

Carbs: 14.7g

Chickpeas and Millet Stew

Preparation Time: 10 minutes

Cooking Time: 1 hour and 5 minutes

Servings: 4

Ingredients:

- 1 cup millet
- 2 tablespoons olive oil
- A pinch of salt and black pepper
- 1 eggplant, cubed
- 1 yellow onion, chopped
- 14 ounces canned tomatoes, chopped
- 14 ounces canned chickpeas, drained and rinsed
- 3 garlic cloves, minced
- 2 tablespoons harissa paste
- 1 bunch cilantro, chopped
- 2 cups water

Directions:

Put the water in a pan, bring to a simmer over medium heat, add the millet, simmer again for about 25 minutes and then take off the heat, fluff with a fork and leave aside for now.

Heat up the pan with half of the oil over medium heat, add the eggplant, salt and pepper, stir, cook for 10 minutes and transfer to a bowl.

Add the rest of the oil to the pan, heat up over medium heat again, add the onion and sauté for 10 minutes.

Add the garlic, more salt and pepper, the harrisa, chickpeas, tomatoes and return the eggplant, stir and then cook in low heat for 15 minutes more.

Add the millet, toss, divide the mix into bowls, sprinkle the cilantro on top and serve.

Nutrition:

Calories: 671

Protein: 27.1

Fat: 15.6

Carbs: 87.5

Crispy Black-Eyed Peas

Preparation Time: 10 minutes

Cooking Time: 15 minutes

Servings: 6

Ingredients:

- 15 ounces black-eyed peas
- 1/8 teaspoon chipotle chili powder
- ¼ teaspoon salt
- ½ teaspoon chili powder
- 1/8 teaspoon black pepper

Directions:

Rinse the beans well with running water then set aside. In a large bowl, mix the spices until well combined. Add the peas to spices and mix. Place the peas in the wire basket and cook for

10 minutes at 360° F. Serve and enjoy!

Nutrition:

Calories: 276

Fat: 9.4 g

Carbs: 8.6 g

Protein: 9.2 g

Lemony Green Beans

Preparation Time: 12 minutes

Cooking Time: 15 minutes

Servings: 4

Ingredients:

- 1 lb. green beans washed and destemmed
- Sea salt and black pepper to taste
- 1 lemon
- ¼ teaspoon extra virgin olive oil

Directions:

Preheat your air fryer to 400°F. Put the green beans in the air fryer basket. Squeeze lemon over beans and season with salt and pepper. Cover ingredients with oil and toss well. Cook green beans for 12 minutes and serve!

Nutrition:

Calories: 263

Fat: 9.2 g

Carbs: 8.6 g

Protein: 8.7 g

Roasted Orange Cauliflower

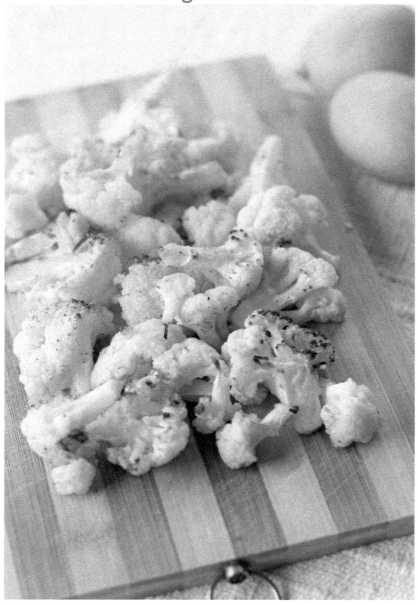

Preparation Time: 20 minutes

Cooking Time: 15 minutes

Servings: 2

Ingredients:

232

- 1 head cauliflower
- ½ lemon, juiced
- ½ tablespoon olive oil
- 1 teaspoon curry powder
- Sea salt and black pepper to taste

Directions:

Prepare your cauliflower by washing and removing the leaves and core. Slice it into florets of comparable size. Grease your air fryer with oil and preheat it for 2 minutes at 390° F. Combine fresh lemon juice and curry powder, add the cauliflower florets and stir. Use salt and pepper as seasoning and stir again. Cook for 20 minutes and serve warm.

Nutrition:

Calories: 263

Fat: 9.2 g

Carbs: 8.6 g

Protein: 8.7 g

Eggplant Parmesan Panini

Preparation Time: 25 minutes

Cooking Time: 15 minutes

Servings: 2

Ingredients:

- 1 medium eggplant, cut into ½ inch slices
- ½ cup mayonnaise
- 2 tablespoons milk
- Black pepper to taste
- ½ teaspoon garlic powder
- ½ teaspoon onion powder
- 1 tablespoon dried parsley
- ½ teaspoon Italian seasoning
- ½ cup breadcrumbs
- Sea salt to taste
- Fresh basil, chopped for garnishing
- ¾ cup tomato sauce
- 2 tablespoons parmesan, grated cheese
- 2 cups grated mozzarella cheese
- 2 tablespoons olive oil
- 4 slices artisan Italian bread
- Cooking spray

Directions:

Cover both sides of eggplant with salt. Place them between sheets of paper towels. Set aside for 30 minutes to get rid of excess moisture. In a mixing bowl, combine Italian seasoning, breadcrumbs, parsley, onion powder, garlic powder and season with salt and pepper. In another small bowl, whisk mayonnaise and milk until smooth.

Preheat your air fryer to 400° F. Remove the excess salt from eggplant slices. Cover both sides of eggplant with mayonnaise mixture. Press the eggplant slices into the breadcrumb mixture. Use cooking spray on both sides of eggplant slices. Air fry slices in batches for 15 minutes, turning over when halfway done. Each bread slice must be greased with olive oil. On a cutting board, place two slices of bread with oiled sides down. Layer mozzarella cheese and grated parmesan cheese. Place eggplant on cheese. Cover with tomato sauce and add remaining mozzarella and parmesan cheeses. Garnish with chopped fresh basil. Put the second slice of bread oiled side up on top. Take preheated Panini press and place sandwiches on it. Close the lid and then cook for about 10 minutes. Slice panini into halves and serve.

Nutrition:

Calories: 267

Fat: 11.3 g

Carbs: 8.7 g

Protein: 8.5 g

Spinach Samosa

Preparation Time: 15 minutes

Cooking Time: 15 minutes

Servings: 2

Ingredients:

- 1 ½ cups of almond flour
- ½ teaspoon baking soda
- 1 teaspoon garam masala
- 1 teaspoon coriander, chopped
- ¼ cup green peas
- ½ teaspoon sesame seeds
- ¼ cup potatoes, boiled, small chunks
- 2 tablespoons olive oil
- ¾ cup boiled and blended spinach puree
- Salt and chili powder to taste

Directions:

In a bowl, mix baking soda, salt, and flour to make the dough. Add 1 tablespoon of oil. Add the spinach puree and mix until the dough is smooth. Place in fridge for 20 minutes. In the pan add one tablespoon of oil, then add potatoes, peas and cook for 5 minutes. Add the sesame seeds, garam masala, coriander, and stir. Knead the dough and make the small ball using a rolling pin. Form balls, make into cone shapes, which are then filled with stuffing that is not yet fully cooked. Make sure flour sheets are well sealed. Preheat air fryer to 390° F. Place samosa in air fryer basket and cook for 10 minutes.

Nutrition:

Calories: 254

Fat: 12.2 g

Carbs: 9.3 g

Protein: 10.2 g

Avocado Fries

Preparation Time: 10 minutes

Cooking Time: 15 minutes

Servings: 4

Ingredients:

- 1 ounce Aquafina
- 1 avocado, sliced
- ½ teaspoon salt
- ½ cup panko breadcrumbs

Directions:

Toss the panko breadcrumbs and salt together in a bowl. Pour Aquafina into another bowl. Dredge the avocado slices in Aquafina and then panko breadcrumbs. Arrange the slices in single layer in air fryer basket. Air fry at 390° F for 10 minutes.

Nutrition:

Calories: 263

Fat: 7.4 g

Carbs: 6.5 g

Protein: 8.2 g

Potato Tortilla with Leeks and Mushrooms

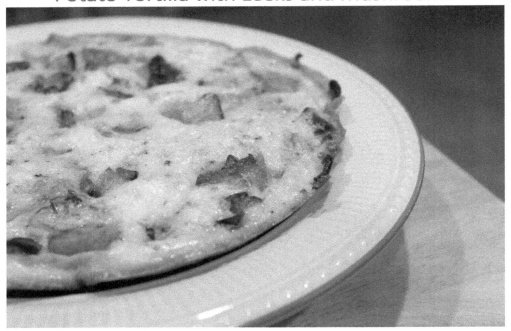

Preparation time: 30 minutes

Cooking time: 50 minutes

Servings: 2

Ingredients:

- 1 tbsp olive oil
- 1 cup leeks, thinly sliced
- 4 ounces baby Bella (cremini) mushrooms, sliced
- 1 small potato, sliced
- 5 large eggs, beaten
- ½ cup unsweetened almond milk
- 1 tsp Dijon mustard
- ½ tsp dried thyme
- ½ tsp salt
- Pinch freshly ground black pepper
- 3 ounces (85 g) Gruyere cheese, shredded

Directions:

1. Prepare the oven to 350 F.
2. Warm-up the olive oil in a pan over medium-high heat.
3. Put the leeks, mushrooms plus potato slices and sauté until the leeks are golden and the potatoes start to brown, about 10 minutes.
4. Adjust to medium-low, cover, and allow the vegetables to cook again within 10 minutes.
5. In the meantime, mix the beaten eggs, milk, mustard, thyme, salt, pepper, plus cheese in a bowl.
6. Move the cooked vegetables to an oiled ovenproof pan and arrange them in a nice layer along the bottom and slightly up the pan's sides.
7. Put the egg batter over the vegetables, then lightly shake to distribute the eggs evenly through the vegetables.
8. Bake within 25 to 30 minutes, remove and cool for 5 minutes before cutting and serving.

Nutrition:

Calories: 541

Fat: 33.1g

Protein: 32.8g

Carbs: 31.0g

Fiber: 4.0g

Sodium: 912mg

Creamy Sweet Potatoes and Collards

Preparation time: 20 minutes

Cooking time: 35 minutes

Servings: 2

Ingredients:

- 1 tablespoon avocado oil

- 3 garlic cloves, chopped

- 1 yellow onion, diced

- ½ teaspoon crushed red pepper flakes

- 1 large sweet potato, peeled and diced

- 2 bunches collard greens (about 2 pounds/907 g), stemmed, leaves chopped into 1-inch squares

- 1 (14.5-ounce / 411-g) can diced tomatoes with juice

- 1 (15-ounce / 425-g) can red kidney beans or chickpeas, drained and rinsed

- 1½ cups water

- ½ cup unsweetened coconut milk

- Salt and black pepper, to taste

Directions:

1. Melt the avocado oil in a large, deep skillet over medium heat.

2. Add the garlic, onion, and red pepper flakes and cook for 3 minutes. Stir in the sweet potato and collards.

3. Add the tomatoes with their juice, beans, water, and coconut milk and mix well. Bring the mixture just to a boil.

4. Reduce the heat to medium-low, cover, and simmer for about 30 minutes, or until softened.

5. Season to taste with salt and pepper and serve.

Nutrition:

Calories: 445

Fat: 9.6g

Protein: 18.1g

Carbs: 73.1g

Fiber: 22.

Sodium: 703mg

Roasted Vegetables and Chickpeas

Preparation time: 15 minutes

Cooking time: 30 minutes

Servings: 2

Ingredients:

- 4 cups cauliflower florets

- 2 medium carrots, sliced into quarters

- 2 tbsp olive oil, divided

- ½ tsp garlic powder, divided

- ½ tsp salt, divided

- 2 tsp zaatar spice mix, divided

- 1 can chickpeas, patted dry

- ¾ cup plain Greek yogurt

- 1 tsp harissa spice paste

Directions:

1. Warm-up, the oven to 400 F. Arrange a sheet pan with parchment paper.

2. Put the cauliflower plus carrots in a bowl, add 1 tablespoon olive oil, ¼ teaspoon of garlic powder, ¼ teaspoon of salt, and 1 teaspoon zaatar. Toss well to combine.

3. Put the vegetables onto half of the sheet pan in a single layer.

4. Put the chickpeas in the same bowl and season with the remaining 1 tablespoon of oil, ¼ teaspoon of garlic powder, and ¼ teaspoon of salt, and the remaining za'atar. Toss well to combine.

5. Put the chickpeas onto the other half of the sheet pan.

6. Roast within 30 minutes. Flip it halfway through the cooking time, and stir the chickpeas, so they cook evenly.

7. In the meantime, mix the yogurt plus harissa in a bowl. Then serve.

Nutrition:

Calories: 468

Fat: 23.0g

Protein: 18.1g

Carbs: 54.1g

Fiber: 13.8g

Sodium: 631mg

Veggie Rice Bowls with Pesto Sauce

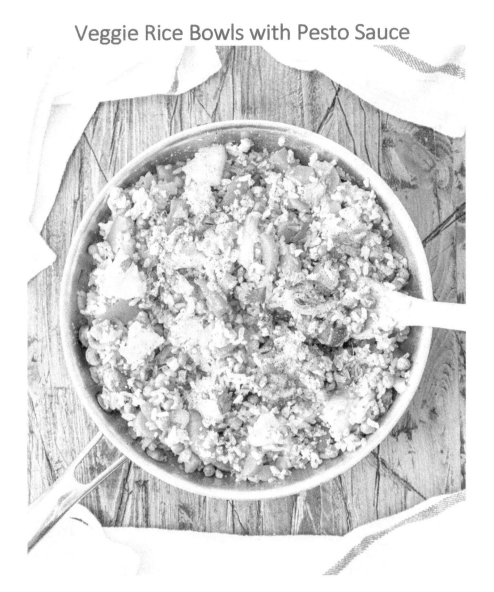

Preparation time: 15 minutes

Cooking time: 1 minute

Servings: 2

Ingredients:

- 2 cups of water

- 1 cup arborio rice, rinsed

- Salt and ground black pepper, to taste

- 2 eggs

- 1 cup broccoli florets

- ½ pound (227 g) Brussels sprouts

- 1 carrot, peeled and chopped

- 1 small beet, peeled and cubed

- ¼ cup pesto sauce

- Lemon wedges, for serving

Directions:

1. Combine the water, rice, salt, and pepper in the Instant Pot. Insert a trivet over rice and place a steamer basket on top.

2. Add the eggs, broccoli, Brussels sprouts, carrots, beet cubes, salt, and pepper to the steamer basket.

3. Lock the lid. Select the Manual mode and set the cooking time for 1 minute at High Pressure.

4. When the timer beeps, perform a natural pressure release for 10 minutes, then release any remaining pressure. Carefully open the lid.

5. Remove the steamer basket and trivet from the pot and transfer the eggs to a bowl of ice water. Peel and halve the eggs. Use a fork to fluff the rice.

6. Divide the rice, broccoli, Brussels sprouts, carrot, beet cubes, and eggs into two bowls. Top with a dollop of pesto sauce and serve with the lemon wedges.

Nutrition:

Calories: 590

Fat: 34.1g

Protein: 21.9g

Carbs: 50.0g

Fiber: 19.6g

Sodium: 670mg

Vegetables

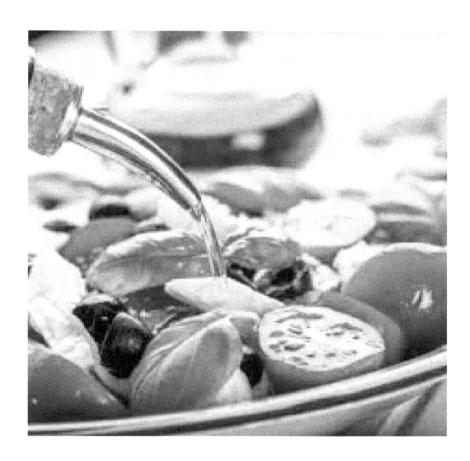

Quinoa with Almonds and Cranberries

Preparation time: 15 minutes

Cooking time: 0 minutes

Servings: 4

Ingredients:

- 2 cups cooked quinoa
- 1/3 teaspoon cranberries or currants
- ¼ cup sliced almonds
- 2 garlic cloves, minced
- 1¼ teaspoons salt
- ½ teaspoon ground cumin
- ½ teaspoon turmeric
- ¼ teaspoon ground cinnamon
- ¼ teaspoon freshly ground black pepper

Directions:

1. In a large bowl, toss the quinoa, cranberries, almonds, garlic, salt, cumin, turmeric, cinnamon, and pepper and stir to combine. Enjoy alone or with roasted cauliflower.

Nutrition:

Calories: 194

Protein: 7g

Carbohydrates: 31g

Sugars: <1g

Fiber: 4g

Fat: 6g

Mediterranean Baked Chickpeas

Preparation time: 15 minutes

Cooking time: 50 minutes

Servings: 4

Ingredients:

- 1 tablespoon extra-virgin olive oil
- ½ medium onion, chopped
- 3 garlic cloves, chopped
- 2 teaspoons smoked paprika
- ¼ teaspoon ground cumin
- 4 cups halved cherry tomatoes
- 2 (15-ounce) cans chickpeas, drained and rinsed
- ½ cup plain, unsweetened, full-fat Greek yogurt, for serving
- 1 cup crumbled feta, for serving

Directions:

1. Preheat the oven to 425 F.

2. In an oven-safe sauté pan or skillet, heat the oil over medium heat and sauté the onion and garlic.

3. Cook within 5 minutes, until softened and fragrant. Mix in the paprika plus cumin and cook for 2 minutes. Stir in the tomatoes and chickpeas.

4. Bring to a simmer for 5 to 10 minutes before placing in the oven. Roast in the oven for 25 to 30 minutes, until bubbling and thickened. To serve, top with Greek yogurt and feta.

Nutrition:

Calories: 412

Protein: 20g

Carbohydrates: 51g

Sugars: 7g

Fiber: 13g

Fat: 15g

Falafel Bites

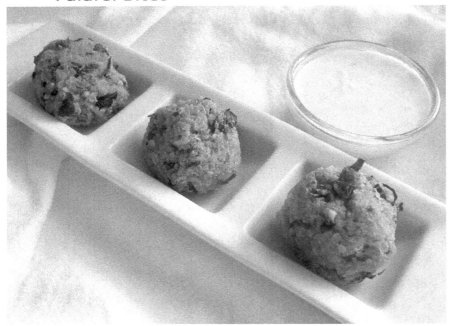

Preparation time: 15 minutes

Cooking time: 10 minutes

Servings: 4

Ingredients:

- 1 2/3 cups falafel mix

- 1¼ cups water

- Extra-virgin olive oil spray

- 1 tablespoon Pickled Onions (optional)

- 1 tablespoon Pickled Turnips (optional)

- 2 tablespoons Tzatziki Sauce (optional)

Directions:

1. In a large bowl, carefully stir the falafel mix into the water. Set aside within 15 minutes to absorb the water. Form the mixture into 1-inch balls and arrange them on a baking sheet.

2. Preheat the broiler to high. Take the balls and flatten slightly with your thumb (so they won't roll around on the baking sheet).

3. Spray with olive oil and then broil for 2 to 3 minutes on each side until crispy and brown.

4. To fry the falafel, fill a pot with ½ inch of cooking oil and heat over medium-high heat to 375°F.

5. Fry the balls within 3 minutes, until brown and crisp. Pat-dry and serve with pickled onions, pickled turnips, and tzatziki sauce (if using).

Nutrition:

Calories: 166

Protein: 17g

Carbohydrates: 30g

Sugars: 5g

Fiber: 8g

Fat: 2g

Quick Vegetable Kebabs

Preparation time: 15 minutes

Cooking time: 15 minutes

Servings: 4

Ingredients:

- 4 medium red onions, sliced into 6 wedges
- 4 medium zucchinis, cut into 1-inch-thick slices
- 4 bell peppers, cut into 2-inch squares
- 2 yellow bell peppers, 2-inch squares
- 2 orange bell peppers, cut into 2-inch squares
- 2 beefsteak tomatoes, cut into quarters
- 3 tablespoons Herbed Oil

Directions:

1. Preheat the oven or grill to medium-high or 350°F. Thread 1-piece red onion, zucchini, different colored bell peppers, and tomatoes onto a skewer.

2. Repeat until the skewer is full of vegetables, up to 2 inches away from the skewer end, and continue until all skewers are complete.

3. Cook in the oven within 10 minutes or grill for 5 minutes on each side. The vegetables will be done with they reach your desired crunch or softness.

4. Remove the skewers from heat and drizzle with Herbed Oil.

Nutrition:

Calories: 240

Protein: 6g

Carbohydrates: 34g

Sugars: 15g

Fiber: 9g

Fat: 12g

Freekeh, Chickpea, and Herb Salad

Preparation time: 15 minutes

Cooking time: 0 minutes

Servings: 6

Ingredients:

- 1 (15-ounce) can chickpeas, rinsed and drained
- 1 cup cooked freekeh
- 1 cup thinly sliced celery
- 1 bunch scallions, chopped
- ½ cup chopped fresh flat-leaf parsley
- ¼ cup chopped fresh mint
- 3 tablespoons chopped celery leaves
- ½ teaspoon kosher salt
- 1/3 cup extra-virgin olive oil
- ¼ cup freshly squeezed lemon juice
- ¼ teaspoon cumin seeds
- 1 teaspoon garlic powder

Directions:

1. In a large bowl, combine the chickpeas, freekeh, celery, scallions, parsley, mint, celery leaves, and salt and toss lightly.

2. Mix the olive oil, lemon juice, cumin seeds, and garlic powder in a small bowl. Once combined, add to freekeh salad.

Nutrition:

Calories: 350

Protein: 9g

Carbohydrates: 38g

Sugars: 1g

Fiber: 9g

Fat: 19g

Mediterranean Farro Bowl

Preparation time: 15 minutes

Cooking time: 10 minutes

Servings: 6

Ingredients:

- 1/3 cup extra-virgin olive oil
- ½ cup chopped red bell pepper
- 1/3 cup chopped red onions
- 2 garlic cloves, minced
- 1 cup zucchini, cut into ½-inch slices
- ½ cup canned chickpeas drained and rinsed
- ½ cup coarsely chopped artichokes
- 3 cups cooked farro
- Salt
- Freshly ground black pepper

For Serving:

- ¼ cup sliced olives (optional)
- ½ cup crumbled feta cheese (optional)
- 2 tablespoons fresh basil, chiffonade (optional)
- 3 tablespoons balsamic reduction (optional)

Directions:

1. In a large sauté pan or skillet, heat the oil over medium heat and sauté the pepper, onions, and garlic for about 5 minutes, until tender.
2. Add the zucchini, chickpeas, and artichokes, then stir and continue to sauté vegetables, approximately 5 more minutes, until just soft.
3. Stir in the cooked farro, tossing to combine and cooking enough to heat through. Put salt plus pepper and remove from the heat.
4. Transfer the contents of the pan into the serving vessels or bowls.

Nutrition:

Calories: 367

Protein: 9g

Carbohydrates: 51g

Sugars: 2g

Fiber: 9g

Fat: 20g

Mozzarella and Sun-Dried Portobello Mushroom Pizza

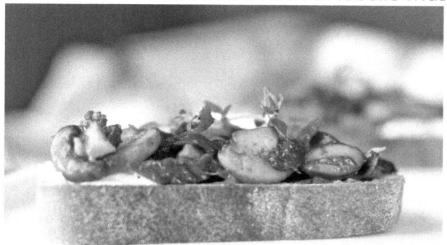

Preparation time: 15 minutes

Cooking time: 10 minutes

Servings: 4

Ingredients:

- 4 large portobello mushroom caps

- 3 tablespoons extra-virgin olive oil

- Salt

- Freshly ground black pepper

- 4 sun-dried tomatoes

- 1 cup mozzarella cheese, divided

- ½ to ¾ cup low-sodium tomato sauce

Directions:

1. Preheat the broiler on high.

2. On a baking sheet, drizzle the mushroom caps with the olive oil and season with salt and pepper. Broil the portobello mushrooms for 5 minutes on each side, flipping once, until tender.

3. Fill each mushroom cap with 1 sun-dried tomato, 2 tablespoons of cheese, and 2 to 3 tablespoons of sauce.

4. Top each with 2 tablespoons of cheese. Place the caps back under the broiler for a final 2 to 3 minutes, then quarter the mushrooms and serve.

Nutrition:

Calories: 218

Protein: 11g

Carbohydrates: 12g

Sugars: 3g

Fiber: 2g

Fat: 16g

Honey Roasted Carrots

Preparation Time: 12 minutes

Cooking Time: 15 minutes

Servings: 2

Ingredients:

- 1 tablespoon honey
- Salt and pepper to taste
- 3 cups of baby carrots
- 1 tablespoon olive oil

Directions:

In a mixing bowl, combine carrots, honey, and olive oil. Season with salt and pepper. Cook in air fryer at 390° F for 12 minutes.

Nutrition:

Calories: 257

Fat: 11.6 g

Carbs: 8.7 g

Protein: 7.3 g

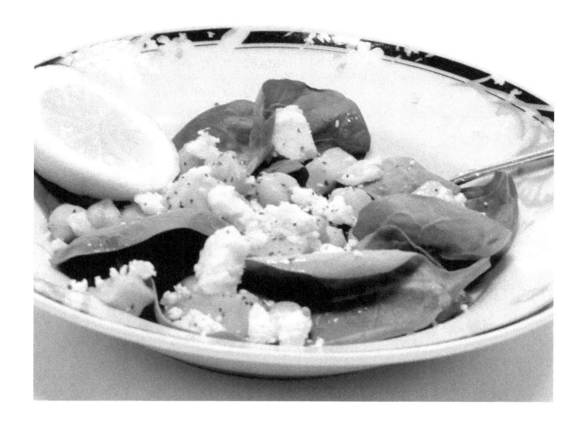

Bacon Cheddar Broccoli Salad

Preparation Time: 35 minutes

Cooking Time: 1 hour

Servings: 6

Ingredients:

- 6 slices raw bacon, chopped
- 1 bunch steamed broccoli, cut into small florets
- ¾ c. mayonnaise
- 2 tbsps. apple cider vinegar
- 3 packets stevia powder
- ½ c. cheddar cheese
- ¼ c. onion, chopped
- ¼ c. sunflower seeds, roasted

Directions:

Take a parchment paper on the bottom of the Crockpot. Take the bacon in the Crockpot.

Cook on low forabout 8 hours until the bacon is crispy.

Take the bacon in a bowl and add the steamed broccoli.

In another bowl, add the mayonnaise, apple cider vinegar, and stevia powder. Mix until well mixed.

Pour over the bacon and broccoli and toss to mix.

Add the cheddar cheese, onion, and sunflower seeds.

Nutrition:

Calories: 345

Carbohydrates: 8.1g

Protein: 16g

Fat: 15.3g

Peppers and Lentils Salad

Preparation time: 10 minutes

Cooking time: 0 minutes

Servings: 4

Ingredients:

- 14 ounces canned lentils, drained and rinsed
- 2 spring onions, chopped
- 1 red bell pepper, chopped
- 1 green bell pepper, chopped
- 1 tablespoon fresh lime juice
- 1/3 cup coriander, chopped
- 2 teaspoon balsamic vinegar

Directions:

1. In a salad bowl, combine the lentils with the onions, bell peppers, and the rest of the ingredients, toss and serve.

Nutrition:

Calories 200

Fat 2.45g

Fiber 6.7g

Carbs 10.5g

Protein 5.6g

Cashews and Red Cabbage Salad

Preparation time: 10 minutes

Cooking time: 0 minutes

Servings: 4

Ingredients:

- 1-pound red cabbage, shredded

- 2 tablespoons coriander, chopped

- ½ cup cashews halved

- 2 tablespoons olive oil

- 1 tomato, cubed

- A pinch of salt and black pepper

- 1 tablespoon white vinegar

Directions:

1. Mix the cabbage with the coriander and the rest of the ingredients in a salad bowl, toss and serve cold.

Nutrition:

Calories 210

Fat 6.3g

Fiber 5.2g

Carbs 5.5g

Protein 8g

Apples and Pomegranate Salad

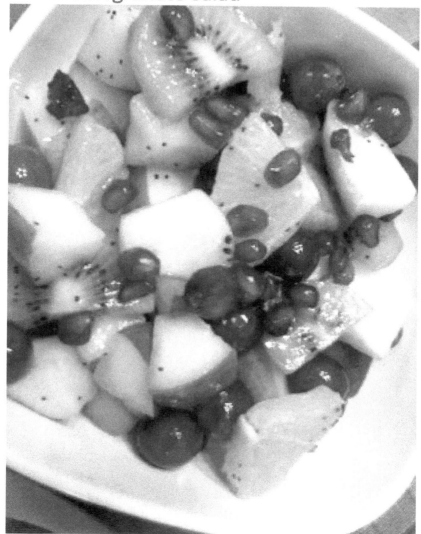

Preparation time: 10 minutes

Cooking time: 0 minutes

Servings: 4

Ingredients:

- 3 big apples, cored and cubed

- 1 cup pomegranate seeds

- 3 cups baby arugula

- 1 cup walnuts, chopped

- 1 tablespoon olive oil

- 1 teaspoon white sesame seeds

- 2 tablespoons apple cider vinegar

- Salt and black pepper to the taste

Directions:

1. Mix the apples with the arugula and the rest of the ingredients in a bowl, toss and serve cold.

Nutrition:

Calories 160

Fat 4.3g

Fiber 5.3g

Carbs 8.7g

Protein 10g

Cranberry Bulgur Mix

Preparation time: 10 minutes

Cooking time: 0 minutes

Servings: 4

Ingredients:

- 1 and ½ cups hot water
- 1 cup bulgur
- Juice of ½ lemon
- 4 tablespoons cilantro, chopped
- ½ cup cranberries, chopped
- 1 and ½ teaspoons curry powder
- ¼ cup green onions, chopped
- ½ cup red bell peppers, chopped
- ½ cup carrots, grated
- 1 tablespoon olive oil
- A pinch of salt and black pepper

Directions:

1. Put bulgur into a bowl, add the water, stir, cover, leave aside for 10 minutes, fluff with a fork, and transfer to a bowl. Add the rest of the ingredients, toss, and serve cold.

Nutrition:

Calories 300

Fat 6.4g

Fiber 6.1g

Carbs 7.6g

Protein 13g

Chickpeas, Corn and Black Beans Salad

Preparation time: 10 minutes

Cooking time: 0 minutes

Servings: 4

Ingredients:

- 1 and ½ cups canned black beans, drained and rinsed
- ½ teaspoon garlic powder
- 2 teaspoons chili powder
- A pinch of sea salt
- black pepper
- 1 and ½ cups canned chickpeas, drained and rinsed
- 1 cup baby spinach
- 1 avocado, pitted, peeled, and chopped
- 1 cup corn kernels, chopped
- 2 tablespoons lemon juice
- 1 tablespoon olive oil
- 1 tablespoon apple cider vinegar
- 1 teaspoon chives, chopped

Directions:

1. Mix the black beans with the garlic powder, chili powder, and the rest of the ingredients in a bowl, toss and serve cold.

Nutrition:

Calories 300

Fat 13.4g

Fiber 4.1g

Carbs 8.6g

Protein 13g

Olives and Lentils Salad

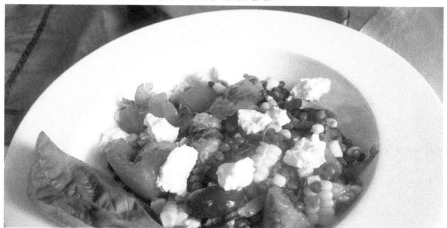

Preparation time: 10 minutes

Cooking time: 0 minutes

Servings: 2

Ingredients:

- 1/3 cup canned green lentils, drained and rinsed
- 1 tablespoon olive oil
- 2 cups baby spinach
- 1 cup black olives, pitted and halved
- 2 tablespoons sunflower seeds
- 1 tablespoon Dijon mustard
- 2 tablespoons balsamic vinegar
- 2 tablespoons olive oil

Directions:

1. Mix the lentils with the spinach, olives, and the rest of the ingredients in a salad bowl, toss and serve cold.

Nutrition:

Calories 279

Fat 6.5g

Fiber 4.5g

Carbs 9.6g

Protein 12g

Lime Spinach and Chickpeas Salad

Preparation time: 10 minutes

Cooking time: 0 minutes

Servings: 4

Ingredients:

- 16 ounces canned chickpeas, drained and rinsed
- 2 cups baby spinach leaves
- ½ tablespoon lime juice
- 2 tablespoons olive oil
- 1 teaspoon cumin, ground
- A pinch of sea salt
- black pepper
- ½ teaspoon chili flakes

Directions:

1. Mix the chickpeas with the spinach and the rest of the ingredients in a large bowl, toss and serve cold.

Nutrition:

calories 240

fat 8.2g

fiber 5.3g

carbs 11.6g

protein 12g

Minty Olives and Tomatoes Salad

Preparation time: 10 minutes

Cooking time: 0 minutes

Servings: 4

Ingredients:

- 1 cup kalamata olives, pitted and sliced
- 1 cup black olives, pitted and halved
- 1 cup cherry tomatoes, halved
- 4 tomatoes, chopped
- 1 red onion, chopped
- 2 tablespoons oregano, chopped
- 1 tablespoon mint, chopped
- 2 tablespoons balsamic vinegar
- ¼ cup olive oil
- 2 teaspoons Italian herbs, dried
- A pinch of sea salt
- black pepper

Directions:

1. In a salad bowl, mix the olives with the tomatoes and the rest of the ingredients, toss, and serve cold.

Nutrition:

Calories 190

Fat 8.1g

Fiber 5.8g

Carbs 11.6g

Protein 4.6g

Beans and Cucumber Salad

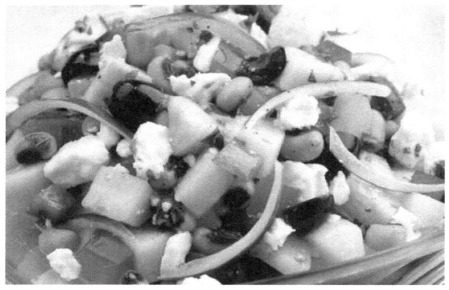

Preparation time: 10 minutes

Cooking time: 0 minutes

Servings: 4

Ingredients:

- 15 oz canned great northern beans
- 2 tablespoons olive oil
- ½ cup baby arugula
- 1 cup cucumber, sliced
- 1 tablespoon parsley, chopped
- 2 tomatoes, cubed
- A pinch of sea salt
- black pepper

- 2 tablespoon balsamic vinegar

Directions:

1. Mix the beans with the cucumber and the rest of the ingredients in a large bowl, toss and serve cold.

Nutrition:

calories 233

fat 9g

fiber 6.5g

carbs 13g

protein 8g

Tomato and Avocado Salad

Preparation time: 10 minutes

Cooking time: 0 minutes

Servings: 4

Ingredients:

- 1-pound cherry tomatoes, cubed

- 2 avocados, pitted, peeled, and cubed

- 1 sweet onion, chopped

- A pinch of sea salt

- black pepper

- 2 tablespoons lemon juice

- 1 and ½ tablespoons olive oil

- Handful basil, chopped

Directions:

1. Mix the tomatoes with the avocados and the rest of the ingredients in a serving bowl, toss and serve right away.

Nutrition:

Calories 148

Fat 7.8g

Fiber 2.9g

Carbs 5.4g

Protein 5.5g

Arugula Salad

Preparation time: 5 minutes

Cooking time: 0 minutes

Servings: 4

Ingredients:

- Arugula leaves (4 cups)
- Cherry tomatoes (1 cup)
- Pine nuts (.25 cup)
- Rice vinegar (1 tbsp.)
- Olive/grapeseed oil (2 tbsp.)
- Grated parmesan cheese (.25 cup)
- Black pepper & salt (as desired)
- Large sliced avocado (1)

Directions:

1. Peel and slice the avocado. Rinse and dry the arugula leaves, grate the cheese, and slice the cherry tomatoes into halves.
2. Combine the arugula, pine nuts, tomatoes, oil, vinegar, salt, pepper, and cheese.
3. Toss the salad to mix and portion it onto plates with the avocado slices to serve.

Nutrition:

Calories: 257

Fats: 23.2 g

Carbohydrates: 10 g

Fiber: 5.9 g

Protein: 6.2 g

Chickpea Salad

Preparation time: 15 minutes

Cooking time: 0 minutes

Servings: 4

Ingredients:

- Cooked chickpeas (15 oz.)

- Diced Roma tomato (1)

- Diced green medium bell pepper (half of 1)

- Fresh parsley (1 tbsp.)

- Small white onion (1)

- Minced garlic (.5 tsp.)

- Lemon (1 juiced)

Directions:

1. Chop the tomato, green pepper, and onion. Mince the garlic. Combine each of the fixings into a salad bowl and toss well.

2. Cover the salad to chill for at least 15 minutes in the fridge. Serve when ready.

Nutrition:

Calories: 163

Fats: 7 g

Carbohydrates: 22 g

Content: 5 g

Protein: 4 g

Feta Tomato Salad

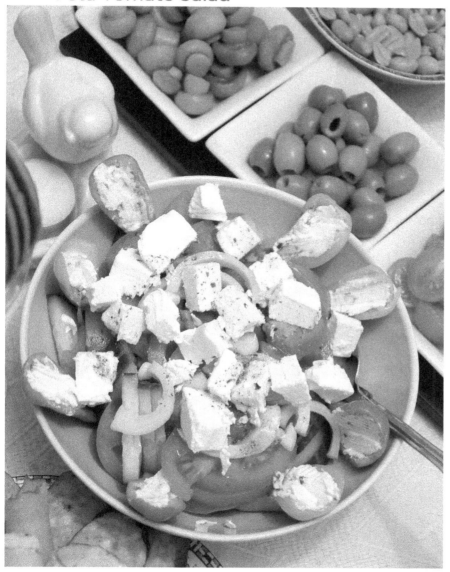

Preparation time: 5 minutes

Cooking time: 0 minutes

Servings: 4

Ingredients:

- Balsamic vinegar (2 tbsp.)

- Freshly minced basil (1.5 tsp.) or Dried (.5 tsp.)

- Salt (.5 tsp.)

- Coarsely chopped sweet onion (.5 cup)

- Olive oil (2 tbsp.)

- Cherry or grape tomatoes (1 lb.)

- Crumbled feta cheese (.25 cup.)

Directions:

1. Whisk the salt, basil, and vinegar. Toss the onion into the vinegar mixture, and wait for about five minutes

2. Slice the tomatoes into halves and stir in the tomatoes, feta cheese, and oil to serve.

Nutrition:

Calories: 121

Fats: 9 g

Carbohydrates: 9 g

Fiber: 2 g

Protein: 3 g

Lebanese Lentil Salad with Garlic & Herbs

Preparation time: 15 minutes

Cooking time: 40 minutes

Servings: 6

Ingredients:

- Green lentils (1 cup)
- Olive oil (4 tbsp. or as needed)
- Garlic (10-12)
- Fresh mint (.75 cup)
- Fresh parsley (.75 cup)
- Ground allspice (.25 tsp.)
- Fresh-squeezed lemon juice (4 tbsp.)
- Ground cumin (1.5 tsp.)
- Freshly cracked black pepper & salt (as desired)

Directions:

1. Remove any stones or broken lentils and rinse them thoroughly. Pour them into a saucepan with three cups of water. Wait for it to boil, then simmer gently until lentils are tender (25-30 min.).
2. While the lentils cook, mince the cloves of garlic. Warm two to three tablespoons of olive oil in a skillet. Toss in the garlic and sauté using low heat (7-8 min.). Turn off the heat.
3. Finely chop the mint and parsley. Whisk the lemon juice, two tablespoons of oil, cumin, and allspice.
4. When lentils are tender, drain the liquids, and dump them into a mixing container.
5. Reheat the garlic pan and pour in the lemon juice dressing mixture to heat it for about one minute.
6. Add the dressing with the lentils, fresh herbs, salt, and pepper. Serve the salad either hot or at room temperature.
7. Serve it for up to two days with a spritz of fresh lemon juice - served at room temperature.

Nutrition:

Calories: 18

Fats: 1 g

Carbs: 21 g

Fiber: 10 g

Protein: 1 g

Lime & Honey Fruit Salad

Preparation time: 5 minutes

Cooking time: 0 minutes

Servings: 8

Ingredients:

- Sliced bananas (2 large)

- Fresh blueberries (.5 lb.)

- Fresh strawberries (1 lb.)

- Honey (2 tbsp.)

- Lime (1 juiced)

- Pine nuts (.33 cup)

Directions:

1. Hull and slice the strawberries and bananas. Combine the blueberries, strawberries, and bananas in a bowl.

2. Drizzle them with the lime juice and honey. Stir well and sprinkle with the nuts before serving.

Nutrition:

Calories: 115

Fats: 3.3 g

Carbohydrates: 22.3 g

Fiber: 3.2 g

Protein: 2.4 g

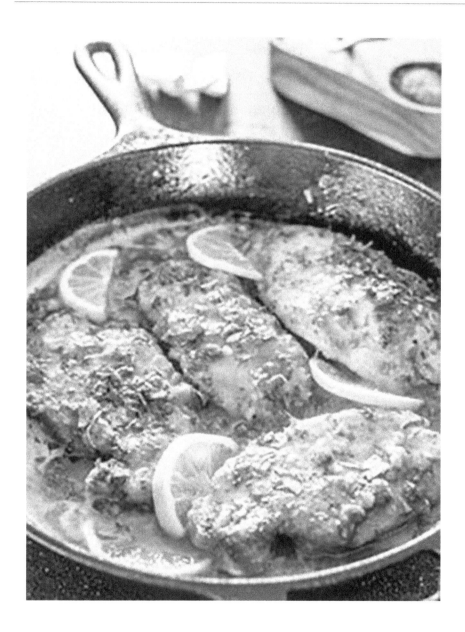

Italian Chicken with Zucchini Noodles

Preparation Time: 1 hour and 10 minutes

Cooking Time: 6 hours

Servings: 6

Ingredients:

- ½ c. chicken broth
- 1 tsp. Italian seasoning
- 4 tsps. tomato paste
- 1-pound chicken breast
- 2 tomatoes, chopped
- 1 ½ c. asparagus
- 1 c. snap peas, halved
- Pepper and salt to taste
- 4 zucchini noodles, cut into noodle-like strips
- 1 c. commercial pesto
- Parmesan cheese for garnish
- Basil for garnish

Directions:

Take the chicken broth, Italian seasoning, tomato paste, chicken breasts, tomatoes, asparagus, and peas in the Crockpot. Give a swirl and season with pepper and salt to

Close the lid and then cook on low for 6 hours. Let it cool before assembling.

Assemble the noodles by placing the chicken mixture on top of the zucchini noodles. Add commercial pesto and garnish with parmesan cheese and basil leaves.

Nutrition:

Calories: 429.7

Carbohydrates: 6g

Protein: 32g

Fat: 26g

Chicken and Kale Tortilla Stew

Preparation Time: 55 minutes

Cooking Time: 5 hours

Servings: 6

Ingredients:

- 4 c. of kale, stems removed and chopped
- 1 tsp. cumin powder
- 6 c. chicken broth
- 2 tbsps. chili powder
- 2 large chicken breasts
- 1 tsp. paprika
- 1 can crushed tomatoes
- 2 tsps. garlic powder
- 1 can sweet corn
- ¼ c. lime juice, freshly squeezed
- ¼ c. Greek yogurt
- 1 can green chilies
- 2 tbsps. minced garlic

Directions:

Take all ingredients except the Greek yogurt in the Crockpot.

Give a stir to mix all ingredients.

Cook on low for 5 hours.

Add the Greek yogurt and continue cooking on high for another hour.

Nutrition:

Calories: 362

Carbohydrates: 10g

Protein: 25g

Fat: 10g

Sticky Chicken Wings

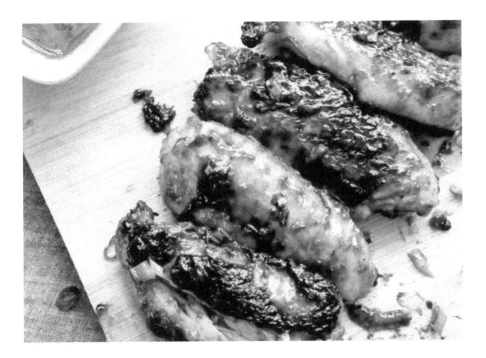

Preparation Time: 20 minutes

Cooking Time: 6 hours

Servings: 6

Ingredients:

- ¼ tsp. salt
- 2 tbsps. Chinese five-spice powder
- 3 tbsps. coconut aminos
- 1 tsp. sesame oil
- ¾ tsp. red pepper flakes
- 1 tbsp. ginger, minced
- 2 tbsps. garlic, minced

- 1 tbsp. xanthan gum

- 3 pounds chicken wings

- Toasted sesame seeds for garnish

Directions:

Mix all ingredients except the sesame seeds.

Stir to coat the chicken wings.

Cook on low for 6 hours.

Garnish with sesame seeds.

Nutrition:

Calories: 475

Carbohydrates: 3g

Protein: 31.8g

Fat: 21g

Lemon Grass and Coconut Chicken Drumsticks

Preparation Time: 15 minutes

Cooking Time: 8 hours

Servings: 6

Ingredients:

- 10 drumsticks, skin removed
- Pepper and salt to taste
- 1 stalk lemongrass, cut into 5-inches long sticks
- 3 tbsps. coconut aminos
- 3 tbsp. EVOO
- 1 thumb-size ginger
- 1 large onion, sliced thinly
- 4 cloves of garlic, minced
- 2 tbsps. fish sauce
- ¼ c. fresh scallions, chopped
- 1 c. coconut milk
- 1 tsp. five-spice powder

Directions:

Take the chicken drumstick in a bowl and season with pepper and salt. Set aside.

In a blender, take the lemongrass, oil ginger, garlic, fish sauce, coconut milk, aminos, and five-spice powder. Blend until a smooth paste is formed.

Pour the paste or sauce into the marinated chicken and mix well. Allow to marinate for another 2 hours.

Take the onion in the Crockpot and add the marinated chicken.

Cook on low for 8 hours.

Sprinkle with scallions on top.

Nutrition:

Calories: 528

Carbohydrates: 2g

Protein: 32g

Fat: 27g

284

Lemon-Rosemary Spatchcock Chicken

Preparation Time: 20 minutes

Cooking Time: 45 minutes

Servings: 6-8

Ingredients:

- ½ cup extra-virgin olive oil, divided
- 1 (3- to 4-pound) roasting chicken
- 8 garlic cloves, roughly chopped
- 2 to 4 tablespoons chopped fresh rosemary
- 2 teaspoons salt, divided
- 1 teaspoon freshly ground black pepper, divided
- 2 lemons, thinly sliced

Directions:

Preheat the oven to 425°F.

Pour in 2 tablespoons of olive oil in the bottom of a 9-by-13-inch baking dish or rimmed baking sheet and swirl to coat the bottom.

To spatchcock the bird, place the whole chicken breast-side down on a large work surface. Cut along the backbone, starting at the tail end and working your way up to the neck. Pull apart the two sides, opening up the chicken. Flip it over, breast-side up, pressing down with your hands to flatten the bird. Transfer to the prepared baking dish.

Loosen the skin of the breast and thigh by cutting a small incision and sticking one or two fingers inside to pull the skin away from the meat without removing it.

To prepare the filling, in a small bowl, combine ¼ cup olive oil, garlic, rosemary, 1 teaspoon salt, and ½ teaspoon pepper and whisk together.

Rub the garlic-herb oil evenly under the skin of each breast and each thigh. Add the lemon slices evenly to the same areas.

Add together the remaining 2 tablespoons olive oil, 1 teaspoon salt, and ½ teaspoon pepper and rub over the outside of the chicken.

Place it in the oven, uncovered, and then roast for 45 minutes, or until cooked through and golden brown.

Nutrition:

Calories: 435

Carbohydrates: 2g

Protein: 28g

Fat: 34g

Chicken Yellow Curry

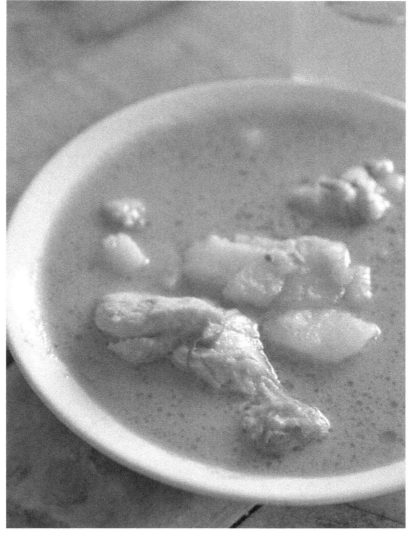

Preparation Time: 40 minutes

Cooking Time: 6 hours

Servings: 6

Ingredients:

- 1 ½ pounds chicken breasts, skin and bones removed
- 6 c. mixed vegetables (preferably broccoli, and cauliflower)

- 1 can full-fat coconut milk
- 2 tsps. ground ginger
- 1 tsp. cinnamon
- 1 c. water
- 2 tsps. ground coriander
- 2 tsps. ground ginger powder
- 1 c. crushed tomatoes
- ½ tsp. cayenne pepper
- 1 tbsp. cumin
- Salt to taste

Directions:

Take the chicken and vegetables in the Crockpot.

Add the rest of the ingredients and stir to mix everything.

Close the lid and then cook on low for 6 hours.

Nutrition:

Calories: 425

Carbohydrates: 3g

Protein: 23g

Fat: 31.4g

Caprese-Stuffed Chicken Breasts

Preparation Time: 20 minutes

Cooking Time: 40 minutes

Servings: 4

Ingredients:

- 8 tablespoons extra-virgin olive oil
- 2 boneless and skinless chicken breasts that are about 6 ounces each
- 4 ounces frozen spinach, thawed and drained well
- 1 cup shredded fresh mozzarella cheese
- ¼ cup chopped fresh basil
- 2 tablespoons chopped sun-dried tomatoes (preferably marinated in oil)
- 1 teaspoon salt, divided
- 1 teaspoon freshly ground black pepper, divided
- ½ teaspoon garlic powder
- 1 tablespoon balsamic vinegar

Directions:

Preheat the oven to 375°F.

Put in 1 tablespoon of olive oil in a small deep baking dish and swirl to coat the bottom.

Make a deep incision about 3- to 4-inches long along the length of each chicken breast to create a pocket. Using your knife or fingers, carefully increase the size of the pocket without cutting through the chicken breast. (Each breast will look like a change purse with an opening at the top.)

In a medium bowl, combine the spinach, mozzarella, basil, sun-dried tomatoes, 2 tablespoons olive oil, ½ teaspoon salt, ½ teaspoon pepper, and the garlic powder and combine well with a fork.

Stuff half of the filling mixture into the pocket of each chicken breast, stuffing down to fully fill the pocket. Press the opening together with your fingers. You can use a couple toothpicks to pin it closed if you wish.

In a medium skillet, heat 2 tablespoons olive oil over medium-high heat. Carefully sear the chicken breasts until browned, 3 to 4 minutes per side, being careful not to let too much filling escape. Transfer to the prepared baking dish, incision-side up. Scrape up any filling that fell out in the skillet and add it to baking dish. Cover the pan with a foil and then bake until the chicken is cooked through, 30-40 minutes depending on the breasts.

Remove it from the oven and et it rest, covered, for 10 minutes. Add together the remaining 3 tablespoons of olive oil, balsamic vinegar, ½ teaspoon salt, and ½ teaspoon pepper.

To serve, cut each chicken breast in half, widthwise, and serve a half chicken breast drizzled with oil and vinegar.

Nutrition:

Calories: 434

Carbohydrates: 3g

Protein: 27g

Fat: 35g

Chicken with Caper Sauce

Preparation Time: *20 minutes*

Cooking Time: *18 minutes*

Servings: 5

Ingredients:

For Chicken:

- 2 eggs
- Salt and ground black pepper, as required
- 1 cup dry breadcrumbs
- 2 tablespoons olive oil
- 1½ pounds skinless, boneless chicken breast halves, pounded into ¾-inch thickness and cut into pieces

For Capers Sauce:

- 3 tablespoons capers
- ½ cup dry white wine
- 3 tablespoons fresh lemon juice
- Salt and ground black pepper, as required
- 2 tablespoons fresh parsley, chopped

Directions:

For chicken: in a shallow dish, add the eggs, salt and black pepper and beat until well combined.

In another shallow dish, place breadcrumbs.

Dip the chicken pieces in egg mixture then coat with the breadcrumbs evenly.

Shake off the excess breadcrumbs.

In a large skillet, heat the oil over medium heat and cook the chicken pieces for about 5-7 minutes per side or until desired doneness.

With a slotted spoon, transfer the chicken pieces onto a paper towel-lined plate.

With a piece of the foil, cover the chicken pieces to keep them warm.

In the same skillet, add all the sauce ingredients except parsley and cook for about 2-3 minutes, stirring continuously.

Stir in the parsley and remove from heat.

Serve the chicken pieces with the topping of capers sauce.

Nutrition:

Calories 352

Total Fat 13.5 g

Saturated Fat 3.5 g

Cholesterol 144 mg

Total Carbs 16.9 g

Sugar 1.9 g

Fiber 1.2 g

Sodium 419 mg

Potassium 111 mg

Protein 35.7 g

Chicken Stuffed Peppers

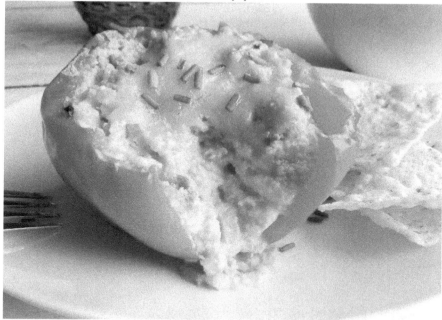

Preparation Time: 10 minutes

Cooking Time: 0 minutes

Servings: 6

Ingredients:

- 1 cup Greek yogurt
- 2 tablespoons mustard
- Salt and black pepper to the taste
- 1-pound rotisserie chicken meat, cubed
- 4 celery stalks, chopped
- 2 tablespoons balsamic vinegar
- 1 bunch scallions, sliced
- ¼ cup parsley, chopped
- 1 cucumber, sliced

- 3 red bell peppers, halved and deseeded
- 1 pint cherry tomatoes, quartered

Directions:

In a bowl, mix the chicken with the celery and the rest of the ingredients except the bell peppers and toss well.

Stuff the peppers halves with the chicken mix and serve for lunch.

Nutrition:

Calories: 266

Protein: 3.7

Fat: 12.2

Carbs: 15.7

Italian Chicken

Preparation Time: 30 minutes

Cooking Time: 10 minutes

Servings: 6

Ingredients:

- 1 carrot, chopped
- 1/2 lb. mushrooms
- 8 chicken thighs
- 1 cup tomato sauce
- 3 cloves garlic, crushed

Directions:

Season the chicken with salt and pepper.

Cover and marinate for 30 minutes.

Press the sauté setting in the Instant Pot.

Add 1 tablespoon of ghee.

Cook the carrots and mushrooms until soft.

Add the tomato sauce and garlic.

Add the chicken, tomatoes and olives.

Cook and mix well.

Seal the pot.

Set it to manual.

Cook at high pressure for 10 minutes.

Release the pressure naturally.

Nutrition:

Calories 425

Total Fat 16.9g

Saturated Fat 5.3g

Cholesterol 179mg

Sodium 395mg

Total Carbohydrate 7.5g

Dietary Fiber 2.1g

Total Sugars 4.5g

Protein 58.9g

Potassium 929mg

Lemon Garlic Chicken

Preparation Time: 1 hour

Cooking Time: 20 minutes

Servings: 6

Ingredients:

- 6 chicken breast fillets
- 3 tablespoons olive oil
- 1 tablespoon lemon juice
- 3 cloves garlic, crushed and minced
- 2 teaspoon dried parsley

Directions:

Marinate the chicken breast fillets in a mixture of olive oil, lemon juice, garlic, parsley, and a pinch of salt and pepper.

Let sit for 1 hour covered in the refrigerator.

Press the sauté setting in the Instant Pot.

Pour in the vegetable oil.

Cook the chicken for 5 minutes per side or until fully cooked.

Nutrition:

Calories 341

Total Fat 17.9g

Saturated Fat 4g

Cholesterol 130mg

Sodium 127mg

Total Carbohydrate 0.7g

Dietary Fiber 0.1g

Total Sugars 0.1g

Protein 42.4g

Potassium 368mg

Chicken with Salsa & Cilantro

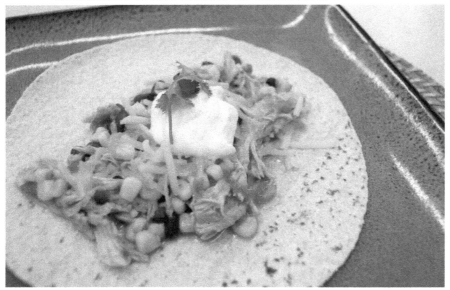

Preparation Time: 20 minutes

Cooking Time: 20 minutes

Servings: 6

Ingredients:

- 1 ½ lb. chicken breast fillets
- 2 cups salsa Verde
- 1 teaspoon garlic, minced
- 1 teaspoon cumin
- 2 tablespoons fresh cilantro, chopped

Directions:

Put the chicken breast fillets inside the Instant Pot.

Pour the salsa, garlic and cumin on top.

Seal the pot.

Set it to poultry.

Release the pressure quickly.

Remove the chicken and shred.

Put it back to the pot.

Stir in the cilantro.

Nutrition:

Calories 238

Total Fat 8.7g

Saturated Fat 2.3g

Cholesterol 101mg

Sodium 558mg

Total Carbohydrate 3.8g

Dietary Fiber 0.4g

Total Sugars 1.2g

Protein 34g

Potassium 285mg

Chicken & Rice

Preparation Time: 20 minutes

Cooking Time: 30 minutes

Servings: 8

Ingredients:

- 1 whole chicken, sliced into smaller pieces.
- 2 tablespoons dry Greek seasoning
- 1 1/2 cups long grain white rice
- 1 cup chopped parsley

Directions:

Coat the chicken with the seasoning mix.

Add 2 cups of water to the Instant Pot.

Add the chicken inside.

Seal the pot.

Choose manual mode.

Cook at high pressure for 30 minutes.

Release the pressure naturally.

Lift the chicken and place on a baking sheet.

Bake in the oven for 5 minutes or until skin is crispy.

While waiting, strain the broth from the Instant Pot to remove the chicken residue.

Add the rice.

Seal the pot.

Set it to rice function.

Fluff the rice and serve with the chicken.

Nutrition:

Calories 412

Total Fat 11.2g

Saturated Fat 3.1g

Cholesterol 130mg

Sodium 249mg

Total Carbohydrate 29.3g

Dietary Fiber 0.7g

Total Sugars 0.1g

Protein 45.1g

Potassium 450mg

Chicken Skillet

Preparation Time: 10 minutes

Cooking Time: 35 minutes

Servings: 6

Ingredients:

- 6 chicken thighs, bone-in and skin-on
- Juice of 2 lemons
- 1 teaspoon oregano, dried
- 1 red onion, chopped
- Salt and black pepper to the taste
- 1 teaspoon garlic powder
- 2 garlic cloves, minced
- 2 tablespoons olive oil
- 2 and ½ cups chicken stock
- 1 cup white rice
- 1 tablespoon oregano, chopped
- 1 cup green olives, pitted and sliced
- 1/3 cup parsley, chopped
- ½ cup feta cheese, crumbled

Directions:

Heat up the pan with the oil in medium heat, add the chicken thighs skin side down, cook it for about 4 minutes in each side and transfer to a plate.

Add the garlic and the onion to the pan, stir and sauté for 5 minutes.

Add the rice, salt, pepper, the stock, oregano, and lemon juice, stir, cook for 1-2 minutes more and take off the heat.

Add the chicken to the pan, introduce the pan in the oven and bake at 375 degrees F for 25 minutes.

Add the cheese, olives and the parsley, divide the whole mix between plates and serve for lunch.

Nutrition:

Calories: 435

Protein: 25.6

Fat: 18.5

Carbs: 27.8

Chicken Shawarma

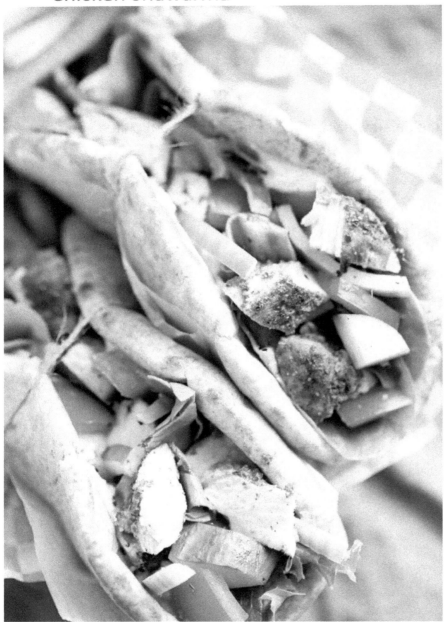

Preparation Time: 15 minutes

Cooking Time: 15 minutes

Servings: 8

Ingredients:

- 2 lb. chicken breast, sliced into strips
- 1 teaspoon paprika
- 1 teaspoon ground cumin
- 1/4 teaspoon granulated garlic
- 1/2 teaspoon turmeric
- 1/4 teaspoon ground allspice

Directions:

Season the chicken with the spices, and a little salt and pepper.

Pour 1 cup chicken broth to the pot.

Seal the pot.

Choose poultry setting.

Cook for 15 minutes.

Release the pressure naturally.

Nutrition:

Calories 132

Total Fat 3g

Saturated Fat 0g

Cholesterol 73mg

Sodium 58mg

Total Carbohydrate 0.5g

Dietary Fiber 0.2g

Total Sugars 0.1g

Protein 24.2g

Potassium 435mg

Mediterranean Chicken

Preparation Time: 10 minutes

Cooking Time: 10 minutes

Servings: 6

Ingredients:

- 2 lb. chicken breast fillet, sliced into strips
- Wine mixture (1/4 cup white wine mixed with 3 tablespoons red wine)
- 2 tablespoons light brown sugar
- 1 1/2 teaspoons dried oregano
- 6 garlic cloves, chopped

Directions:

Pour in the wine mixture to the Instant Pot.

Stir in the rest of the ingredients.

Toss the chicken to coat evenly.

Seal the pot.

Set it to high pressure.

Cook for 10 minutes.

Release the pressure naturally.

Nutrition:

Calories 304

Total Fat 11.3g

Saturated Fat 3.1g

Cholesterol 135mg

Sodium 131mg

Total Carbohydrate 4.2g

Dietary Fiber 0.2g

Total Sugars 3g

Protein 44g

Potassium 390mg

Lime Chicken with Black Beans

Preparation Time: 20 minutes

Cooking Time: 10 minutes

Servings: 8

Ingredients:

- 8 chicken thighs (boneless and skinless)
- 3 tablespoons lime juice
- 1 cup black beans
- 1 cup canned tomatoes
- 4 teaspoons garlic powder

Directions:

Marinate the chicken in a mixture of lime juice and garlic powder.

Add the chicken to the Instant Pot.

Pour the tomatoes on top of the chicken.

Seal the pot.

Set it to manual.

Cook at high pressure for 10 minutes.

Release the pressure naturally.

Stir in the black beans.

Press sauté to simmer until black beans are cooked.

Nutrition:

Calories 370

Total Fat 11.2g

Saturated Fat 3.1g

Cholesterol 130mg

Sodium 128mg

Total Carbohydrate 17.5g

Dietary Fiber 4.1g

Total Sugars 1.5g

Protein 47.9g

Potassium 790mg

Mediterranean Chicken Wings

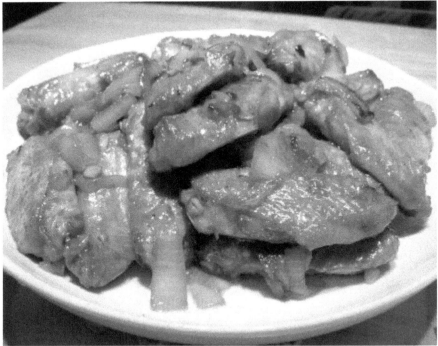

Preparation Time: 1 hour

Cooking Time: 20 minutes

Servings: 4

Ingredients:

- 8 chicken wings
- 1 tablespoon garlic puree
- 2 tablespoons mixed dried herbs (tarragon, oregano and basil)
- 1 tablespoon chicken seasoning

Directions:

In a bowl, mix the garlic puree, herbs and seasoning.

Marinate the chicken in this mixture for 1 hour.

Add 1 tablespoon of coconut oil into the Instant Pot.

Set it to sauté.

Cook the chicken until brown on both sides.

Remove and set aside.

Add 1 cup of water to the pot.

Place steamer basket inside.

Put the chicken on top of the basket.

Seal the pot.

Set it to manual and cook at high pressure for 10 minutes.

Release the pressure naturally.

Nutrition:

Calories 280

Total Fat 11.2g

Saturated Fat 3g

Cholesterol 130mg

Sodium 135mg

Total Sugars 0g

Protein 42.2g

Potassium 355mg

Honey Balsamic Chicken

Preparation Time: 30 minutes

Cooking Time: 20 minutes

Servings: 10

Ingredients:

- 1/4 cup honey
- 1/2 cup balsamic vinegar
- 1/4 cup soy sauce
- 2 cloves garlic minced
- 10 chicken drumsticks

Directions:

Mix the honey, vinegar, soy sauce and garlic in a bowl.

Marinate the chicken in the sauce for 30 minutes.

Cover the pot.

Set it to manual.

Cook at high pressure for 10 minutes.

Release the pressure quickly.

Choose the sauté button to thicken the sauce.

Serving Suggestion: Garnish with lemon wedges.

Tip: You can also use chicken wings or other chicken parts for this recipe.

Nutrition:

Calories 184

Total Fat 4.4g

Saturated Fat 1.2g

Cholesterol 67mg

Sodium 662mg

Total Carbohydrate 13g

Dietary Fiber 0.1g

Total Sugars 11.9g

Protein 21.9g

Potassium 202mg

Turkey Verde with Brown Rice

Preparation Time: 10 minutes

Cooking Time: 24 minutes

Servings: 5

Ingredients:

- 2/3 cup chicken broth
- 1 1/4 cup brown rice
- 1 1/2 lb. turkey tenderloins
- 1 onion, sliced
- 1/2 cup salsa Verde

Directions:

Add the chicken broth and rice to the Instant Pot.

Top with the turkey, onion and salsa.

Cover the pot.

Set it to manual.

Cook at high pressure for 18 minutes.

Release the pressure naturally.

Wait for 8 minutes before opening the pot.

Serving Suggestion: Garnish with fresh cilantro.

Tip: Use long grain brown rice.

Nutrition:

Calories 336

Total Fat 3.3g

Saturated Fat 0.3g

Cholesterol 54mg

Sodium 321mg

Total Carbohydrate 39.4g

Dietary Fiber 2.2g

Total Sugars 1.4g

Protein 38.5g

Potassium 187mg

Turkey with Basil & Tomatoes

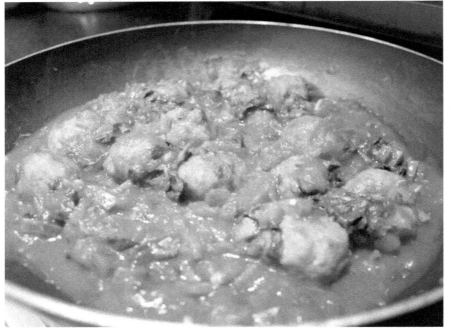

Preparation Time: 10 minutes

Cooking Time: 10 minutes

Servings: 4

Ingredients:

- 4 turkey breast fillets
- 1 tablespoon olive oil
- 1/4 cup fresh basil, chopped
- 1 1/2 cups cherry tomatoes, sliced in half
- 1/4 cup olive tapenade

Directions:

Season the turkey fillets with salt.

Add the olive oil to the Instant Pot.

Set it to sauté.

Cook the turkey until brown on both sides.

Stir in the basil, tomatoes and olive tapenade.

Cook for 3 minutes, stirring frequently.

Serving Suggestion: Serve with green salad.

Tip: Use freshly chopped basil leaves.

Nutrition:

Calories 188

Total Fat 5.1g

Saturated Fat 1g

Cholesterol 0mg

Sodium 3mg

Total Carbohydrate 2.8g

Dietary Fiber 1.6g

Total Sugars 1.9g

Protein 33.2g

Potassium 164mg

Desserts

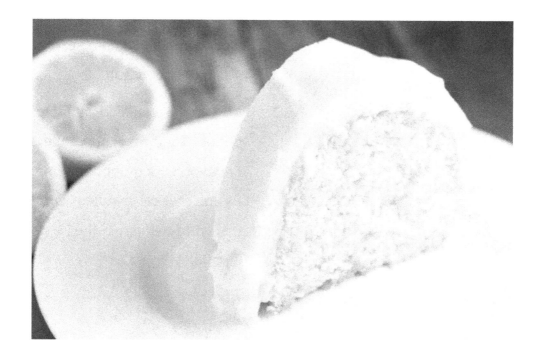

Butter Pie

Preparation Time: 10 minutes

Cooking Time: 15 minutes

Servings: 2

Ingredients:

- 3 whole eggs
- 6 tbsp of all-purpose flour
- 1 ½ cup of milk
- Salt to taste
- 4 tbsp of butter
- 1 cup of skim sour cream
- 1 tbsp of ground red pepper

Directions:

Preheat the oven to 300°. Line in some baking paper over a baking dish and then set it aside.

Mix well three eggs, all-purpose flour, 2 table spoons of butter, milk, and salt.

Spread the mixture on a baking dish and then bake it for about 15 minutes.

When done, remove from the oven and cool for a while. Chop into bite-sized pieces and place on a serving plate. Pour 1 cup of sour cream.

Melt the remaining 2 table spoons of butter over a medium temperature. Add 1 tablespoon of ground red pepper and stir-fry for several minutes. Drizzle some of this mixture over the pie and serve immediately.

Nutrition:

Calories 317

Fat 17g

Carbs 36g

Protein 24g

Homemade Spinach Pie

Preparation Time: 20 minutes

Cooking Time: 30 minutes

Servings: 5

Ingredients:

- lb. fresh spinach
- 0.5 lb. fresh dandelion leaves
- ¼ cup of Feta cheese, crumbled
- ½ cup of sour cream
- ½ cup of blue cheese, chopped
- 2 eggs
- 2 tbsp of butter, melted
- Salt to taste
- 1 pack of pie crust
- Vegetable oil

Directions:

Preheat the oven to 350 degrees. Use 1 table spoon of butter to grease the baking dish. Add the ingredients in a large bowl and then mix well. Grease the pie crust with some oil. Spread the spinach mixture over the pie crust and roll. Place in a baking dish and then bake for about 30-40 minutes

Remove from the heat and serve warm.

Nutrition:

Calories 230

Fat 9g

Carbs 29g

Protein 11g

Blueberries Bowls

Preparation Time: 10 minutes

Cooking Time: 0 minutes

Servings: 4

Ingredients:

- 1 teaspoon vanilla extract

- 2 cups blueberries

- 1 teaspoon coconut sugar

- 8 ounces Greek yogurt

Directions:

1. Mix strawberries with the vanilla and the other **ingredients**, toss and serve cold.

Nutrition:

343 calories

13.4g fat

5.5g protein

Rhubarb Strawberry Crunch

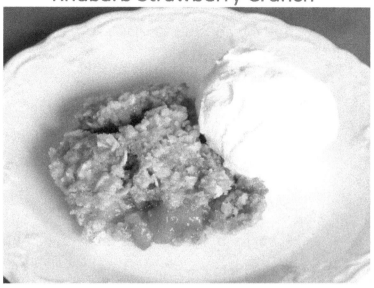

Preparation Time: 20 minutes

Cooking Time: 60 minutes

Servings: 18

Ingredients:

- 3 tbsps. all-purpose flour
- 3 c. fresh strawberries, sliced
- 3 c. rhubarb, cubed
- 1 ½ c. flour
- 1 c. packed brown sugar
- 1 c. butter
- 1 c. oatmeal

Directions:

Preheat the oven to 374°F

In a medium bowl mix rhubarb, 3 tbsps flour, white sugar, and strawberries. Set the mixture in a baking dish.

In another bowl mix 1 ½ cups of flour, brown sugar, butter, and oats until a crumbly texture is obtained. You may use a blender.

Combine mixtures and place on the baking pan

Bake for 45 minutes or until crispy and light brown.

Nutrition:

Calories 253

Fat 10.8g

Carbs 38.1g

Protein 2.3g

Banana Dessert with Chocolate Chips

Preparation Time: 20 minutes

Cooking Time: 30 minutes

Servings: 24

Ingredients:

- 2/3 c. white sugar
- ¾ c. butter
- 2/3 c. brown sugar
- 1 egg, beaten
- 1 tsp. vanilla extract
- 1 c. banana puree
- 1 ¾ c. flour
- 2 tsps. baking powder
- ½ tsp. salt
- 1 c. semi-sweet chocolate chips

Directions:

Preheat oven at 350°F

In a bowl, add the sugars and butter and beat until lightly colored

Add the egg and vanilla.

Add the banana puree and stir

In another bowl mix baking powder, flour, and salt. Add this mixture to the butter mixture

Stir in the chocolate chips

Prepare a baking pan and place the dough onto it

Bake for 20 minutes and let it cool for 5 minutes before slicing into equal squares

Nutrition:

Calories 174

Fat 8.2g

Carbs 25.2g

Protein 1.7g

Cranberry and Pistachio Biscotti

Preparation Time: 20 minutes

Cooking Time: 60 minutes

Servings: 4

Ingredients:

- ¼ c. light olive oil
- ¾ c. white sugar
- 2 tsps. vanilla extract
- ½ tsp. almond extract
- 2 eggs
- 1 ¾ c. all-purpose flour
- ¼ tsp. salt
- 1 tsp. baking powder
- ½ c. dried cranberries
- 1 ½ c. pistachio nuts

Directions:

Preheat the oven at 300 F/ 148 C

Combine olive oil and sugar in a bowl and mix well

Add eggs, almond and vanilla extracts, stir

Add baking powder, salt, and flour

Add cranberries and nuts, mix

Divide the dough in half — form two 12 x 2-inch logs on a parchment baking sheet.

Set in the oven and bake for 35 minutes or until the blocks are golden brown. Set from oven and allow to cool for about 10 minutes.

Set the oven to 275 F/ 135 C

Cut diagonal trunks into 3/4-inch-thick slices. Place on the sides on the baking sheet covered with parchment

Bake for about 8 - 10 minutes or until dry

You can serve it both hot and cold

Nutrition:

Calories 92

Fat 4.3g

Carbs 11.7g

Protein 2.1g

Minty Watermelon Salad

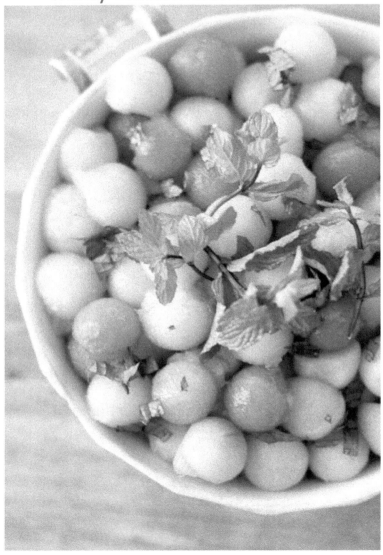

Preparation Time: 10 minutes

Cooking Time: None

Servings: 6-8

Ingredients:

- 1 medium watermelon
- 1 cup fresh blueberries
- 2 tablespoons fresh mint leaves
- 2 tablespoons lemon juice
- ⅓ cup honey

Directions:

Cut the watermelon into 1-inch cubes. Put them in a bowl.

Evenly distribute the blueberries over the watermelon.

Cchop the mint leaves and then put them into a separate bowl.

Add the lemon juice and honey to the mint and whisk together.

Drizzle the mint dressing over the watermelon and blueberries. Serve cold

Nutrition:

Calories 238

Fat 1g

Carbs 61g

Protein 4g

Mascarpone and Fig Crostini

Preparation Time: 10 minutes

Cooking Time: 10 minutes

Servings: 6-8

Ingredients:

- 1 long French baguette
- 4 tablespoons (½ stick) salted butter, melted
- 1 (8-ounce) tub mascarpone cheese
- 1 (12-ounce) jar fig jam or preserves

Directions:

Preheat the oven to 350°F.

Slice the bread into ¼-inch-thick slices.

Lay out the sliced bread on a single baking sheet and brush each slice with the melted butter.

Put the singleaking sheet in the oven and toast the bread for 5 to 7 minutes, just until golden brown.

Let the bread cool slightly. Spread it about a tea spoon or so of the mascarpone cheese on each piece of bread.

Top with a teaspoon or so of the jam. Serve immediately.

Nutrition:

Calories 445

Fat 24g

Carbs 48g

Protein 3g

Crunchy Sesame Cookies

Preparation Time: 10 minutes

Cooking Time: 15 minutes

Servings: 14-16

Ingredients:

- 1 cup sesame seeds, hulled
- 1 cup sugar
- 8 tablespoons (1 stick) salted butter, softened
- 2 large eggs
- 1¼ cups flour

Directions:

Preheat the oven to 350°F. Toast the sesame seeds on a baking sheet for 3 minutes. Set aside and let cool.

Using a mixer, cream together the sugar and butter.

Put the eggs one at a time until well-blended.

Add the flour and toasted sesame seeds and mix until well-blended.

Drop spoonfuls of cookie dough onto a baking sheet and form them into round balls, about 1-inch in diameter, similar to a walnut.

Put in the oven and bake for 5 to 7 minutes or until golden brown.

Let the cookies cool and enjoy.

Nutrition:

Calories 218

Fat 12g

Carbs 25g

Protein 4g

Almond Cookies

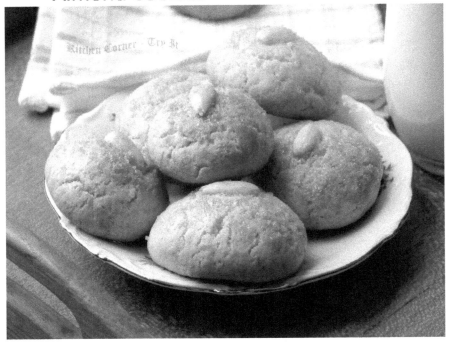

Preparation Time: 5 minutes

Cooking Time: 10 minutes

Servings: 4-6

Ingredients:

- ½ cup sugar
- 8 tablespoons (1 stick) room temperature salted butter
- 1 large egg
- 1½ cups all-purpose flour
- 1 cup ground almonds or almond flour

Directions:

Preheat the oven to 375°F.

Using a mixer, cream together the sugar and butter.

Add the egg and mix until combined.

Alternately add the flour and ground almonds, ½ cup at a time, while the mixer is on slow.

Once everything is combined, line a baking sheet with parchment paper. Drop a tablespoon of dough on the baking sheet, keeping the cookies at least 2 inches apart.

Put the single baking sheet in the oven and bake just until the cookies start to turn brown around the edges for about 5 to 7 minutes.

Nutrition:

Calories 604

Fat 36g

Carbs 63g

Protein 11g

Baklava and Honey

Preparation Time: 40 minutes

Cooking Time: 1 hour

Servings: 6-8

Ingredients:

- 2 cups chopped walnuts or pecans
- 1 teaspoon cinnamon
- 1 cup of melted unsalted butter
- 1 (16-ounce) package phyllo dough, thawed
- 1 (12-ounce) jar honey

Directions:

Preheat the oven to 350°F.

In a bowl, combine the chopped nuts and cinnamon.

Using a brush, butter the sides and bottom of a 9-by-13-inch inch baking dish.

Take off the phyllo dough from the package and cut it to the size of the baking dish using a sharp knife.

Put one sheet of phyllo dough on the bottom of the dish, brush with butter, and repeat until you have 8 layers.

Sprinkle ⅓ cup of the nut mixture over the phyllo layers. Top with a sheet of phyllo dough, butter that sheet, and repeat until you have 4 sheets of buttered phyllo dough.

Sprinkle ⅓ cup of the nut mixture for another layer of nuts. Repeat the layering of nuts and 4 sheets of buttered phyllo until all the nut mixture is gone. The last layer should be 8 buttered sheets of phyllo.

Before you bake, cut the baklava into desired shapes; traditionally this is diamonds, triangles, or squares.

Bake the baklava for about 1 hour just until the top layer is golden brown.

While the baklava is baking, heat the honey in a pan just until it is warm and easy to pour.

Once the baklava is done baking, directly pour the honey evenly over the baklava and let it absorb it, about 20 minutes. Serve warm or at room temperature.

Nutrition:

Calories 1235

Fat 89g

Carbs 109g

Protein 18g

Date and Nut Balls

Preparation Time: 10 minutes

Cooking Time: 10 minutes

Servings: 6-8

Ingredients:

- 1 cup walnuts or pistachios
- 1 cup unsweetened shredded coconut
- 14 medjool dates, pits removed
- 8 tablespoons (1 stick) butter, melted

Directions:

Preheat the oven to 350°F.

Put the nuts on a baking sheet. Toast the nuts for 5 minutes.

Put the shredded coconut on a clean baking sheet; toast just until it turns golden brown, about 3 to 5 minutes (coconut burns fast so keep an eye on it). Once done, remove it from the oven and put it in a shallow bowl.

Inside a food processor with a chopping blade, put the nuts until they have a medium chop. Put the chopped nuts into a medium bowl.

Add the dates and melted butter to the food processor and blend until the dates become a thick paste. Pour the chopped nuts into the food processor with the dates and pulse just until the mixture is combined, about 5 to 7 pulses.

Remove the mixture from the food processor and scrape it into a large bowl.

To make the balls, spoon 1 to 2 tablespoons of the date mixture into the palm of your hand and roll around between your hands until you form a ball. Put the ball on a clean, lined baking sheet. Repeat this until all of the mixture is formed into balls.

Roll each ball in the toasted coconut until the outside of the ball is coated, put the ball back on the baking sheet, and repeat.

Put all the balls into the fridge for 20 minutes before serving so that they firm up. You can also store any leftovers inside the fridge in an airtight container.

Nutrition:

Calories 489

Fat 35g

Carbs 48g

Protein 5g

Creamy Rice Pudding

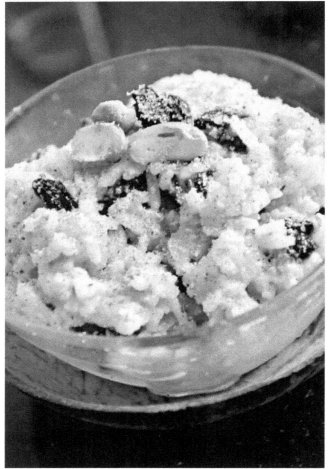

Preparation Time: 5 minutes

Cooking Time: 45 minutes

Servings: 6

Ingredients:

- 1¼ cups long-grain rice
- 5 cups whole milk
- 1 cup sugar
- 1 tablespoon of rose water/orange blossom water

- 1 teaspoon cinnamon

Directions:

Rinse the rice under cold water for 30 seconds.

Add the rice, milk, and sugar in a large pot. Bring to a gentle boil while continually stirring.

Lessen the heat to low and then let simmer for 40 to 45 minutes, stirring every 3 to 4 minutes so that the rice does not stick to the bottom of the pot.

Add the rose water at the end and simmer for 5 minutes.

Divide the pudding into 6 bowls. Sprinkle the top with cinnamon. Let it cool for over an hour before serving. Store in the fridge.

Nutrition:

Calories 394

Fat 7g

Carbs 75g

Protein 9g

Ricotta-Lemon Cheesecake

Preparation Time: 5 minutes

Cooking Time: 1 hour

Servings: 8-10

Ingredients:

- 2 (8-ounce) packages full-fat cream cheese
- 1 (16-ounce) container full-fat ricotta cheese
- 1½ cups granulated sugar
- 1 tablespoon lemon zest
- 5 large eggs
- Nonstick cooking spray

Directions:

Preheat the oven to 350°F.

Blend together the cream cheese and ricotta cheese.

Blend in the sugar and lemon zest.

Blend in the eggs; drop in 1 egg at a time, blend for 10 seconds, and repeat.

Put a 9-inch springform pan with a parchment paper and nonstick spray.

Wrap the bottom of the pan with foil. Pour the cheesecake batter into the pan.

To make a water bath, get a baking or roasting pan larger than the cheesecake pan. Fill the roasting pan about ⅓ of the way up with warm water. Put the cheesecake pan into the water bath. Put the whole thing in the oven and let the cheesecake bake for 1 hour.

After baking is complete, remove the cheesecake pan from the water bath and remove the foil. Let the cheese cake cool for 1 hour on the countertop. Then put it in the fridge to cool for at least 3 hours before serving.

Nutrition:

Calories 489

Fat 31g

Carbs 42g

Protein 15g

Crockpot Keto Chocolate Cake

Preparation Time: 20 minutes

Cooking Time: 3 hours

Servings: 12

Ingredients:

- ¾ c. stevia sweetener
- 1 ½ c. almond flour
- ¼ tsp. baking powder
- ¼ c. protein powder, chocolate, or vanilla flavor
- 2/3 c. unsweetened cocoa powder
- ¼ tsp. salt
- ½ c. unsalted butter, melted
- 4 large eggs
- ¾ c. heavy cream
- 1 tsp. vanilla extract

Directions:

Grease the ceramic insert of the Crockpot.

In a bowl, mix the sweetener, almond flour, protein powder, cocoa powder, salt, and baking powder.

Add the butter, eggs, cream, and vanilla extract.

Pour the batter in the Crockpot and cook on low for 3 hours.

Allow to cool before slicing.

Nutrition:

Calories: 253

Carbohydrates: 5.1g

Protein: 17.3g

Fat: 29.5g

Keto Crockpot Chocolate Lava Cake

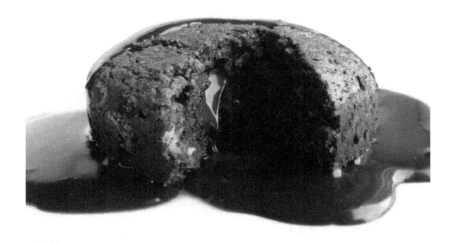

Preparation Time: 30 minutes

Cooking Time: 3 hours

Servings: 12

Ingredients:

- 1 ½ c. stevia sweetener, divided
- ½ c. almond flour
- 5 tbsps. unsweetened cocoa powder
- ½ tsp. salt
- 1 tsp. baking powder
- 3 whole eggs
- 3 egg yolks
- ½ c. butter, melted
- 1 tsp. vanilla extract
- 2 c. hot water

- 4 ounces sugar-free chocolate chips

Directions:

Grease the inside of the Crockpot.

In a bowl, mix the stevia sweetener, almond flour, cocoa powder, salt, and baking powder.

In another bowl, mix the eggs, egg yolks, butter, and vanilla extract. Pour in the hot water.

Pour the wet **ingredients** to the dry **ingredients** and fold to create a batter.

Add the chocolate chips last

Pour into the greased Crockpot and cook on low for 3 hours.

Allow to cool before serving.

Nutrition:

Calories: 157

Carbohydrates: 5.5g

Protein: 10.6g

Fat: 13g

Lemon Crockpot Cake

Preparation Time: 15 minutes

Cooking Time: 3 hours

Servings: 8

Ingredients:

- ½ c. coconut flour
- 1 ½ c. almond flour
- 3 tbsps. stevia sweetener
- 2 tsps. baking powder
- ½ tsp. xanthan gum
- ½ c. whipping cream
- ½ c. butter, melted
- 1 tbsp. juice, freshly squeezed
- Zest from one large lemon
- 2 eggs

Directions:

Grease the inside of the Crockpot with a butter or cooking spray.

Mix together coconut flour, almond flour, stevia, baking powder, and xanthan gum in a bowl.

In another bowl, combine the whipping cream, butter, lemon juice, lemon zest, and eggs. Mix until well combined.

Pour the wet **ingredients** to the dry **ingredients** gradually and fold to create a smooth batter.

Spread the batter in the Crockpot and cook on low for 3 hours

Nutrition:

Calories: 350

Carbohydrates: 11.1g

Protein: 17.6g

Fat: 32.6g

Lemon and Watermelon Granita

Preparation Time: 10 minutes + 3 hours to freeze

Cooking Time: None

Servings: 4

Ingredients:

- 4 cups watermelon cubes
- ¼ cup honey
- ¼ cup freshly squeezed lemon juice

Directions:

In a blender, combine the watermelon, honey, and lemon juice. Purée all the **ingredients**, then pour into a 9-by-9-by-2-inch baking pan and place in the freezer.

Every 30 to 60 minutes, run a fork across the frozen surface to fluff and create ice flakes. Freeze for about 3 hours total and serve.

Nutrition:

Calories: 153

Carbohydrates: 39g

Protein: 2g

Fat: 1g

Baked Apples with Walnuts and Spices

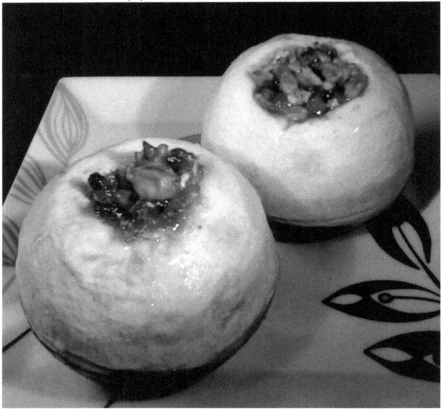

Preparation Time: 10 minutes

Cooking Time: 45 minutes

Servings: 4

Ingredients:

- 4 apples
- ¼ cup chopped walnuts
- 2 tablespoons honey
- 1 teaspoon ground cinnamon
- ¼ teaspoon ground nutmeg
- ¼ teaspoon ground ginger

- Pinch sea salt

Directions:

Preheat the oven to 375°F.

Cut the tops off the apples and then use a metal spoon or a paring knife to remove the cores, leaving the bottoms of the apples intact. Place the apples cut-side up in a 9-by-9-inch baking pan.

Stir together the walnuts, honey, cinnamon, nutmeg, ginger, and sea salt. Put the mixture into the centers of the apples. Bake the apples for about 45 minutes until browned, soft, and fragrant. Serve warm.

Nutrition:

Calories: 199

Carbohydrates: 41g

Protein: 5g

Fat: 5g

Red Wine Poached Pears

Preparation Time: 10 minutes

Cooking Time: 45 minutes + 3 hours to chill

Servings: 4

Ingredients:

- 2 cups dry red wine
- ¼ cup honey
- Zest of ½ orange
- 2 cinnamon sticks
- 1 (1-inch) piece fresh ginger
- 4 pears, bottom inch sliced off so the pear is flat

Directions:

In a pot on medium-high heat, stir together the wine, honey, orange zest, cinnamon, and ginger. Bring to a boil, stirring occasionally. Lessen the heat to medium-low and then simmer for 5 minutes to let the flavors blend.

Add the pears to the pot. Cover and simmer for 20 minutes until the pears are tender, turning every 3 to 4 minutes to ensure even color and contact with the liquid. Refrigerate the pears in the liquid for 3 hours to allow for more flavor absorption.

Bring the pears and liquid to room temperature. Place the pears on individual dishes and return the poaching liquid to the stove top over medium-high heat. Simmer for 15 minutes until the liquid is syrupy. Serve the pears with the liquid drizzled over the top.

Nutrition:

Calories: 283

Carbohydrates: 53g

Protein: 1g

Fat: 1g

Vanilla Pudding with Strawberries

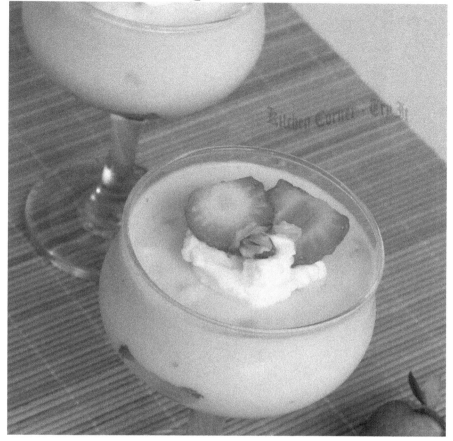

Preparation Time: 10 minutes

Cooking Time: 10 minutes + chilling time

Servings: 4

Ingredients:

- 2¼ cups skim milk, divided
- 1 egg, beaten
- ½ cup sugar
- 1 teaspoon vanilla extract
- Pinch sea salt

- 3 tablespoons cornstarch
- 2 cups sliced strawberries

Directions:

In a small bowl, whisk 2 cups of milk with the egg, sugar, vanilla, and sea salt. Transfer the mixture to a medium pot, place it over medium heat, and slowly bring to a boil, whisking constantly.

Whisk the cornstarch with the ¼ cup of milk. In a thin stream, whisk this slurry into the boiling mixture in the pot. Cook until it thickens, stirring constantly. Boil for 1 minute more, stirring constantly.

Spoon the pudding into 4 dishes and refrigerate to chill. Serve topped with the sliced strawberries.

Nutrition:

Calories: 209

Carbohydrates: 43g

Protein: 6g

Fat: 1g

Mixed Berry Frozen Yogurt Bar

Preparation Time: 10 minutes

Cooking Time: None

Servings: 8

Ingredients:

- 8 cups low-fat vanilla frozen yogurt (or flavor of choice)
- 1 cup sliced fresh strawberries
- 1 cup fresh blueberries
- 1 cup fresh blackberries
- 1 cup fresh raspberries
- ½ cup chopped walnuts

Directions:

Apportion the yogurt among 8 dessert bowls. Serve the toppings family style, and let your guests choose their toppings and spoon them over the yogurt.

Nutrition:

Calories: 81

Carbohydrates: 9g

Protein: 3g

Fat:

Vanilla Cream

Preparation Time: 2 hours

Cooking Time: 10 minutes

Servings: 4

Ingredients:

- 1 cup almond milk
- 1 cup coconut cream
- 2 cups coconut sugar
- 2 tablespoons cinnamon powder
- 1 teaspoon vanilla extract

Directions:

1. Heat up a pan with the almond milk over medium heat, add the rest of the **ingredients**, whisk, and cook for 10 minutes more.

2. Divide the mix into bowls, cool down and keep in the fridge for 2 hours before serving.

Nutrition:

254 calories

7.5g fat

9.5g protein

Brownies

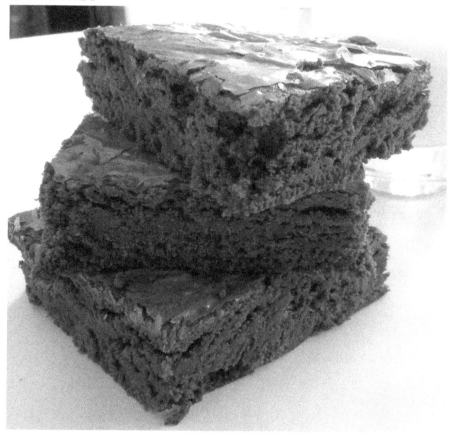

Preparation Time: 10 minutes

Cooking Time: 25 minutes

Servings: 8

Ingredients:

- 1 cup pecans, chopped

- 3 tablespoons coconut sugar

- 2 tablespoons cocoa powder

- 3 eggs, whisked

- ¼ cup avocado oil

- ½ teaspoon baking powder

- 2 teaspoons vanilla extract

- Cooking spray

Directions:

1. In your food processor, combine the pecans with the coconut sugar and the other ingredients except the cooking spray and pulse well.

2. Grease a square pan with cooking spray, add the brownies mix, spread, introduce in the oven, bake at 350 degrees F for 25 minutes, leave aside to cool down, slice and serve.

Nutrition:

370 calories

14.3g fat

5.6g protein

Strawberries Coconut Cake

Preparation Time: 10 minutes

Cooking Time: 25 minutes

Servings: 6

Ingredients:

- 2 cups almond flour
- 1 cup strawberries, chopped
- ½ teaspoon baking soda
- ½ cup coconut sugar
- ¾ cup coconut milk
- ¼ cup avocado oil
- 2 eggs, whisked
- 1 teaspoon vanilla extract
- Cooking spray

Directions:

1. In a bowl, combine the flour with the strawberries and the other ingredients except the cooking spray and whisk well.
2. Grease a cake pan with cooking spray, pour the cake mix, spread, bake in the oven at 350 degrees F for 25 minutes, cool down, slice and serve.

Nutrition:

465 calories

22g fat

13.4g protein

Cocoa Almond Pudding

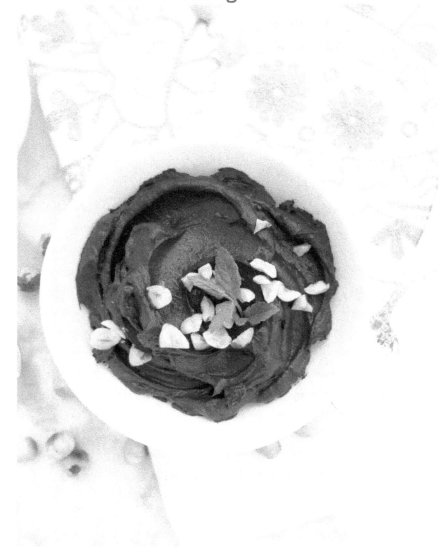

Preparation Time: 10 minutes

Cooking Time: 10 minutes

Servings: 4

Ingredients:

- 2 tablespoons coconut sugar

- 3 tablespoons coconut flour

- 2 tablespoons cocoa powder

- 2 cups almond milk

- 2 eggs, whisked

- ½ teaspoon vanilla extract

Directions:

1. Fill milk in a pan, add the cocoa and the other **ingredients**, whisk, simmer over medium heat for 10 minutes, pour into small cups and serve cold.

Nutrition:

385 calories

31.7g fat

7.3g protein

Nutmeg Cream

Preparation Time: 10 minutes

Cooking Time: 0 minutes

Servings: 6

Ingredients:

- 3 cups almond milk

- 1 teaspoon nutmeg, ground

- 2 teaspoons vanilla extract

- 4 teaspoons coconut sugar

- 1 cup walnuts, chopped

Directions:

1.   In a bowl, combine milk with the nutmeg and the other **ingredients**, whisk well, divide into small cups and serve cold.

Nutrition:

243 calories

12.4g fat

9.7g protein

Vanilla Avocado Cream

Preparation Time: 70 minutes

Cooking Time: 0 minutes

Servings: 4

Ingredients:

- 2 cups coconut cream

- 2 avocados, peeled, pitted and mashed

- 2 tablespoons coconut sugar

- 1 teaspoon vanilla extract

Directions:

1. Blend cream with the avocados and the other **ingredients**, pulse well, divide into cups and keep in the fridge for 1 hour before serving.

Nutrition:

532 calories

48.2g fat

5.2g protein

Raspberries Cream Cheese Bowls

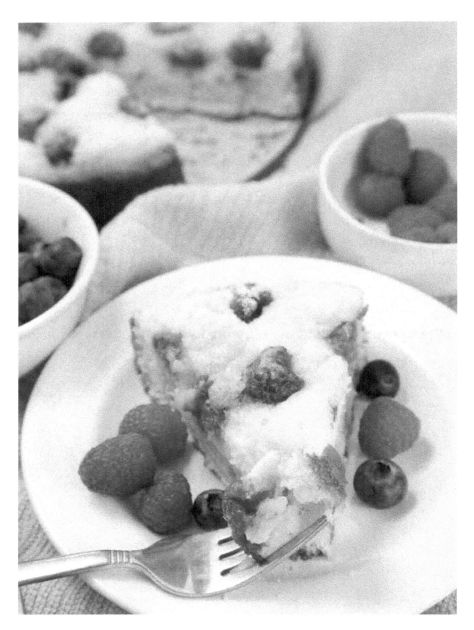

Preparation Time: 10 minutes

Cooking Time: 25 minutes

Servings: 4

354

Ingredients:

- 2 tablespoons almond flour

- 1 cup coconut cream

- 3 cups raspberries

- 1 cup coconut sugar

- 8 ounces cream cheese

Directions:

1.   In a bowl, the flour with the cream and the other **ingredients**, whisk, transfer to a round pan, cook at 360 degrees F for 25 minutes, divide into bowls and serve.

Nutrition:

429 calories

36.3g fat

7.8g protein

Mediterranean Watermelon Salad

Preparation time: 4 minutes

Cooking time: 0 minutes

Servings: 4

Ingredients:

- 1 cup watermelon, peeled and cubed

- 2 apples, cored and cubed

- 1 tablespoon coconut cream

- 2 bananas, cut into chunks

Directions:

1.   Incorporate watermelon with the apples and the other **ingredients**, toss and serve.

Nutrition:

131 calories

1.3g fat

1.3g protein

Coconut Apples

Preparation Time: 10 minutes

Cooking Time: 10 minutes

Servings: 4

Ingredients:

- 2 teaspoons lime juice

- ½ cup coconut cream

- ½ cup coconut, shredded

- 4 apples, cored and cubed

- 4 tablespoons coconut sugar

Directions:

1. Incorporate apples with the lime juice and the other **ingredients**, stir, bring to a simmer over medium heat and cook for 10 minutes.

2. Divide into bowls and serve cold.

Nutrition:

320 calories

7.8g fat

4.7g protein

Orange Compote

Preparation Time: 10 minutes

Cooking Time: 15 minutes

Servings: 4

Ingredients:

- 5 tablespoons coconut sugar

- 2 cups orange juice

- 4 oranges, peeled and cut into segments

Directions:

1.   In a pot, combine oranges with the sugar and the orange juice, toss, bring to a boil over medium heat, cook for 15 minutes, divide into bowls and serve cold.

Nutrition:

220 calories

5.2g fat

5.6g protein

Pears Stew

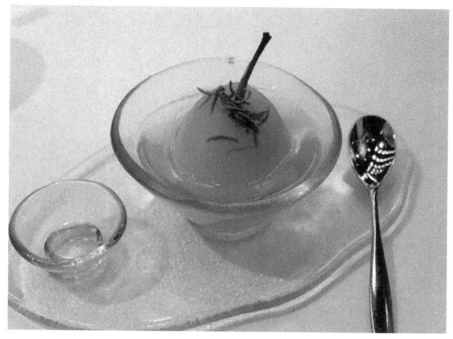

Preparation Time: 10 minutes

Cooking Time: 15 minutes

Servings: 4

Ingredients:

- 2 cups pears, cored and cut into wedges
- 2 cups water
- 2 tablespoons coconut sugar
- 2 tablespoons lemon juice

Directions:

1.   In a pot, combine the pears with the water and the other **ingredients**, toss, cook over medium heat for 15 minutes, divide into bowls and serve.

Nutrition:

260 calories

6.2g fat

6g protein

Lemon Watermelon Mix

Preparation Time: 10 minutes

Cooking Time: 10 minutes

Servings: 4

Ingredients:

- 2 cups watermelon

- 4 tablespoons coconut sugar

- 2 teaspoons vanilla extract

- 2 teaspoons lemon juice

Directions:

1. In a small pan, combine the watermelon with the sugar and the other **ingredients**, toss, heat up over medium heat, cook for about 10 minutes, divide into bowls and serve cold.

Nutrition:

140 calories

4g fat

5g protein

Rhubarb Cream

Preparation Time: 10 minutes

Cooking Time: 14 minutes

Servings: 4

Ingredients:

- 1/3 cup cream cheese

- ½ cup coconut cream

- 2-pound rhubarb, roughly chopped

- 3 tablespoons coconut sugar

Directions:

1. Blend cream cheese with the cream and the other **ingredients** well.

2. Divide into small cups, introduce in the oven and bake at 350 degrees F for 14 minutes.

3. Serve cold.

Nutrition:

360 calories

14.3g fat

5.2g protein

Mango Bowls

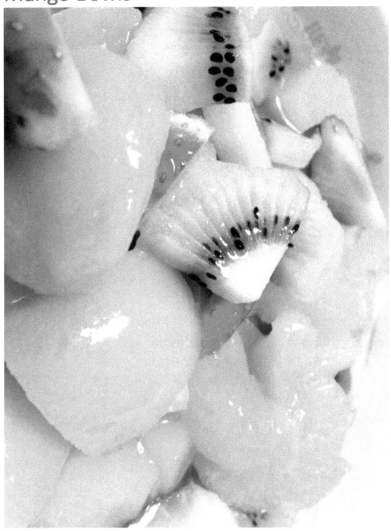

Preparation Time: 10 minutes

Cooking Time: 0 minutes

Servings: 4

Ingredients:

- 3 cups mango, peeled and cubed

- 1 teaspoon chia seeds

- 1 cup coconut cream

- 1 teaspoon vanilla extract

- 1 tablespoon mint, chopped

Directions:

1. Mix mango with the cream and the other **ingredients**, toss, divide into smaller bowls and keep in the fridge for 10 minutes before serving.

Nutrition:

238 calories

16.6g fat

3.3g protein

Chocolate Ganache

Preparation time: 10 minutes

Cooking Time: 16 minutes

Servings: 16

Ingredients

- 9 ounces bittersweet chocolate, chopped

- 1 cup heavy cream

- 1 tablespoon dark rum (optional)

Direction

1. Situate chocolate in a medium bowl. Cook cream in a small saucepan over medium heat.

2. Bring to a boil. When the cream has reached a boiling point, pour the chopped chocolate over it and beat until smooth. Stir the rum if desired.

3. Allow the ganache to cool slightly before you pour it on a cake. Begin in the middle of the cake and work outside. For a fluffy icing or chocolate filling, let it cool until thick and beat with a whisk until light and fluffy.

Nutrition:

142 calories

10.8g fat

1.4g protein

Chocolate Covered Strawberries

Preparation Time: 15 minutes

Cooking Time: 0 minute

Servings: 24

Ingredients

- 16 ounces milk chocolate chips

- 2 tablespoons shortening

- 1-pound fresh strawberries with leaves

Direction

1. In a bain-marie, melt chocolate and shortening, occasionally stirring until smooth. Pierce the tops of the strawberries with toothpicks and immerse them in the chocolate mixture.

2. Turn the strawberries and put the toothpick in Styrofoam so that the chocolate cools.

Nutrition:

115 calories

7.3g fat

1.4g protein

Strawberry Angel Food Dessert

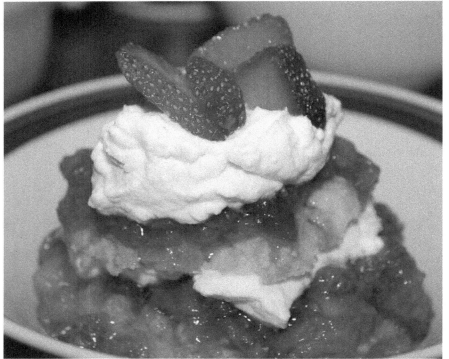

Preparation Time: 15 minutes

Cooking Time: 0 minutes

Servings: 18

Ingredients

- 1 angel cake (10 inches)

- 2 packages of softened cream cheese

- 1 cup of white sugar

- 1 container (8 oz) of frozen fluff, thawed

- 1 liter of fresh strawberries, sliced

- 1 jar of strawberry icing

Direction

1. Crumble the cake in a 9 x 13-inch dish.

2. Beat the cream cheese and sugar in a medium bowl until the mixture is light and fluffy. Stir in the whipped topping. Crush the cake with your hands, and spread the cream cheese mixture over the cake.

3. Combine the strawberries and the frosting in a bowl until the strawberries are well covered. Spread over the layer of cream cheese. Cool until ready to serve.

Nutrition:

261 calories

11g fat

3.2g protein

Fruit Pizza

Preparation Time: 30 minutes

Cooking Time: 0 minute

Servings: 8

Ingredients

- 1 (18-oz) package sugar cookie dough

- 1 (8-oz) package cream cheese, softened

- 1 (8-oz) frozen filling, defrosted

- 2 cups of freshly cut strawberries

- 1/2 cup of white sugar

- 1 pinch of salt

- 1 tablespoon corn flour

- 2 tablespoons lemon juice

- 1/2 cup orange juice

- 1/4 cup water

- 1/2 teaspoon orange zest

Direction

1. Ready oven to 175 ° C Slice the cookie dough then place it on a greased pizza pan. Press the dough flat into the mold. Bake for 10 to 12 minutes. Let cool.

2. Soften the cream cheese in a large bowl and then stir in the whipped topping. Spread over the cooled crust.

3. Start with strawberries cut in half. Situate in a circle around the outer edge. Continue with the fruit of your choice by going to the center. If you use bananas, immerse them in lemon juice. Then make a sauce with a spoon on the fruit.

4. Combine sugar, salt, corn flour, orange juice, lemon juice, and water in a pan. Boil and stir over medium heat. Boil for 1 or 2 minutes until thick. Remove from heat and add the grated orange zest. Place on the fruit.

5. Allow to cool for two hours, cut into quarters, and serve.

Nutrition

535 calories

30g fat

5.5g protein

Bananas Foster

Preparation Time: 5 minutes

Cooking Time: 6 minutes

Servings: 4

Ingredients

- 2/3 cup dark brown sugar
- 1/4 cup butter
- 3 1/2 tablespoons rum
- 1 1/2 teaspoons vanilla extract
- 1/2 teaspoon of ground cinnamon
- 3 bananas, peeled and cut lengthwise and broad
- 1/4 cup coarsely chopped nuts
- vanilla ice cream

Direction

1. Melt the butter in a deep-frying pan over medium heat. Stir in sugar, rum, vanilla, and cinnamon.
2. When the mixture starts to bubble, place the bananas and nuts in the pan. Bake until the bananas are hot, 1 to 2 minutes. Serve immediately with vanilla ice cream.

Nutrition:

534 calories

23.8g fat

4.6g protein

Cranberry Orange Cookies

Preparation Time: 20 minutes

Cooking Time: 16 minutes

Servings: 24

Ingredients

- 1 cup of soft butter
- 1 cup of white sugar
- 1/2 cup brown sugar
- 1 egg
- 1 teaspoon grated orange peel
- 2 tablespoons orange juice
- 2 1/2 cups flour
- 1/2 teaspoon baking powder
- 1/2 teaspoon salt
- 2 cups chopped cranberries
- 1/2 cup chopped walnuts (optional)

Icing:

- 1/2 teaspoon grated orange peel
- 3 tablespoons orange juice
- 1 ½ cup confectioner's sugar

Direction

1. Preheat the oven to 190 ° C.

2. Blend butter, white sugar, and brown sugar. Beat the egg until everything is well mixed. Mix 1 teaspoon of orange zest and 2 tablespoons of orange juice. Mix the flour, baking powder, and salt; stir in the orange mixture.

3. Mix the cranberries and, if used, the nuts until well distributed. Place the dough with a spoon on ungreased baking trays.

4. Bake in the preheated oven for 12 to 14 minutes. Cool on racks.

5. In a small bowl, mix icing **ingredients**. Spread over cooled cookies.

Nutrition:

110 calories

4.8g fat

1.1 g protein

CPSIA information can be obtained
at www.ICGtesting.com
Printed in the USA
BVHW061106030521
606339BV00010B/1397